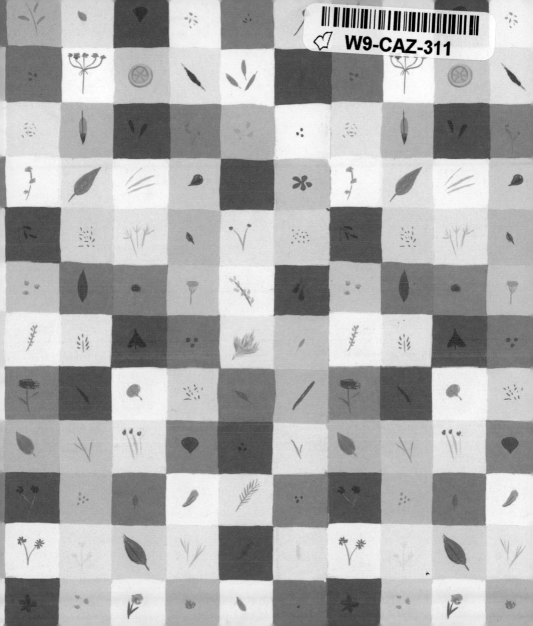

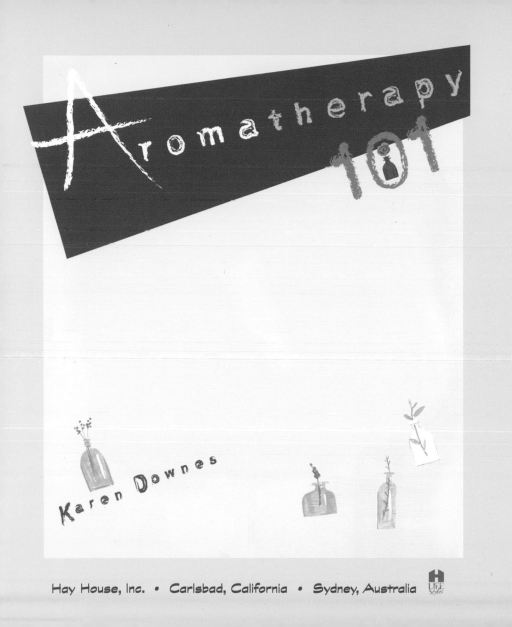

Aromatherapy 101

Karen Downes

Hay House, Inc. • Carlsbad, California • Sydney, Australia

Published and distributed in the United States by:
Hay House, Inc., P.O. Box 5100, Carlsbad, CA 92018-5100
(800) 654-5126 • (800) 650-5115 (fax)

Editorial Supervision: Jill Kramer
Interior Design: Jenny Richards • Illustrations: Juliette Borda

Library of Congress Cataloging-in-Publication Data

Downes, Karen, aromatherapist.
     Aromatherapy 101 / Karen Downes.
          p. cm.
     ISBN 1-561-70692-2 (hardcover)
     1. Aromatherapy-Popular works. I. Title. II. Aromatherapy one hundred and
one. III. Title: Aromatherapy one hundred one.

RM666.A68 D68 2000
615'.321 21-dc21   99-043689

ISBN 1-56170-692-2

03 02 01 00   5 4 3 2
1st printing, May 2000
2nd printing, June 2000

Printed in China by Imago

Contents

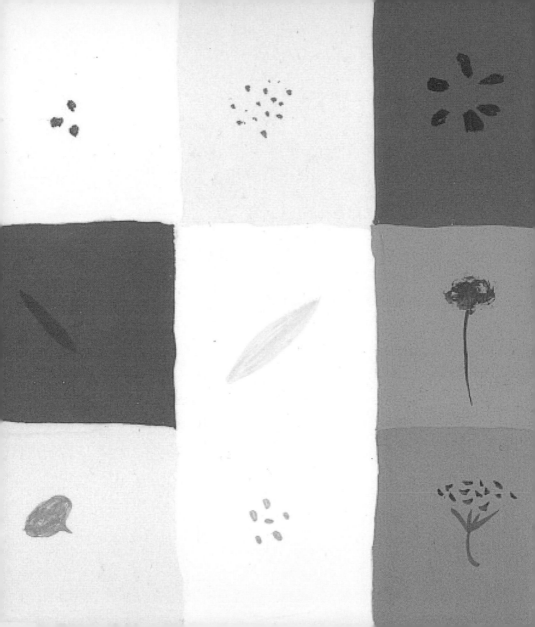

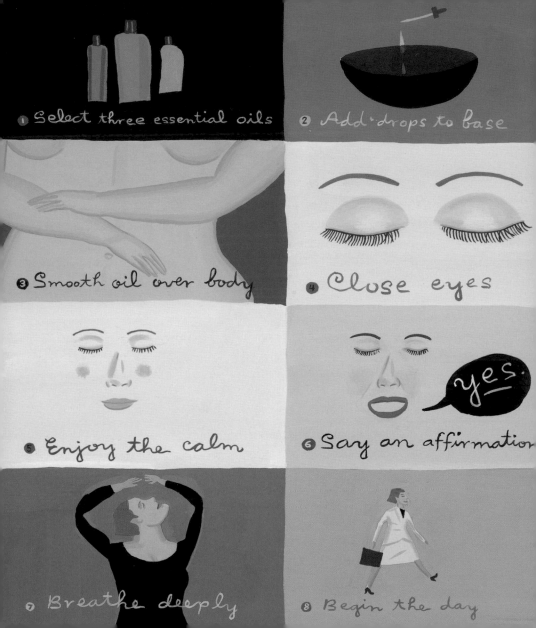

Aromatherapy—What Is It?

As the word implies, *aromatherapy* uses "aromas" to aid healing and well-being—aromas we smell every day in Mother Nature's garden. It's long been known that Mother Nature provides us with an extensive medicine cabinet, and aromatherapy lets us use her gifts in an empowering way. Oil is extracted from her flowers, trees, bushes, and herbs, and is used to treat a wide range of human ailments—in some cases, those of our pets. It's the use of these essential oils in our everyday lives that can uplift our moods and senses, provide first aid, and assist us in getting closer to ourselves through greater awareness.

Essential Oils—What Are They?

The greatest dilemma that many people face today is the speed of change. Coinciding with the dynamics of change is often a sense of separation and isolation. However, there is help at hand.

Since time began, human beings have looked to nature as a resource. The cycle of the seasons can be depended on; the regeneration of plants can be trusted. The medicine provided by thousands of plant species to heal our bodies and minds is at our fingertips with aromatherapy practices. So often, our spirits are rejuvenated by activities such as a walk in the park or a weekend in the country. With the daily use of essential oils, these benefits can now be ex-tended into our personal lives.

As our senses are tantalized, our memories and emotions are evoked, and our bodies seduced into relaxation through the power of the aromatic, volatile plant extracts known as *essential oils*. Knowledge has been handed down through the ages regarding the contributions that essential oils can make in our lives. Some of the stories originated in our grandmothers' tales, some were told by wise sages, while others were revealed by those deeply in touch with the plants. Whichever way the information has reached us, one thing is certain: Essential oils could not have endured the test of time had they not been established and revered as a reliable and resourceful healing modality.

So what exactly are essential oils? An essential oil is a substance extracted from a single botanical source; the extract is 70 times more concentrated than what is originally found in plant form. Being highly aromatic, essential oils are prized in the perfume industry, and the scent also plays an important role in aromatherapy. These volatile substances are found in many different parts of the plant. Orange, for example, is taken from the peel, while Eucalyptus is found in the leaf of the tree.

The process of extraction varies somewhat according to the oil that is being extracted; the most common form is steam distillation. In this process, the plant material is harvested and placed in a large enclosed vat. Then, with enormous pressure, steam is passed through the vat, rupturing the oil-bearing glands of the plant. The aromatic vapor rises and passes through a chamber surrounded by cold water, where the vapor condenses, and, now in a liquid form, separates into water and oil. The essential oil is then removed from the surface of the water.

Essential oils can also be extracted using solvents, as well as by cold pressing. Whichever way they are extracted, it is important to use only pure oils for aromatherapy. Essential oils contain many components that occur naturally in the plant, so it is crucial that they remain "essential" so that they can work for us on the body and in it.

It is the wisdom of Mother Nature that creates each plant's unique chemical combinations. An intellectual process in a laboratory cannot possibly imitate what Mother Nature does intuitively. When practicing aromatherapy, choose your oil with discernment.

Developing Your Wisdom
Knowing How to Choose
Your Essential Oils

In ancient Tibet, ignorance was considered the primary source of all suffering. Aromatherapy awakens our senses and connects us deeply with nature and with the inner message of self-regeneration that is inherent in the plants. As we expand our awareness of what essential oils can do, we deepen our trust in our intuition, which will guide us to the right oils at the right time.

Healing ourselves begins with insight into the source of our distress or our challenge. As we look closely at our lives and what is causing the disturbance, we discover that this is the first step to healing ourselves, and at the same time, to developing our inner wisdom. Thus, we become even more clear that we are our own healers.

Essential oils are at hand to give us what our bodies need. Study the characteristics of each individual oil so that you get to know it, just like you would become acquainted with a dear friend. A great way to do this is to take a new oil each day, dilute it, and apply 1 or 2 drops to a pulse point on your body, such as on the inside of your wrist. Inhale its fragrance deeply, read over its qualities, and throughout the day, take in the aroma and remind yourself of its gifts.

Browse with your nose—use your sense of smell to guide you in the selection process each time you choose your oils, since it is intrinsically linked to your intuition. There are no set guidelines on having to blend this or that—simply choose 3 oils to create your blend. The experiment begins as you dispense the drops into a bath, base oil, or vaporizer. (See Ways to Use Essential Oils on the next page for more information.)

HOW MANY DROPS SHOULD YOU USE?

Essential oils are concentrated substances and should always be used with a gentle hand. For general home use, a combination of 3 essential oils; 8 drops to a bath or vaporizer; or 3 drops to a massage blend is recommended until you have a better understanding of the oils and how to work with them. It's okay to use more drops with the guiding hand of an aromatherapist, or if you have experience with essential oils.

It's important to take note of an oil's toxicity levels (see *Safety Information* in the A-Z rundown of essential oils), and even more important, to know which oils can be used during pregnancy. If you've never used essential oils before and you're pregnant, it's recommended that you wait until after the birth of your child before you start using them. Additionally, people with sensitive skin should take extra care when using all essential oils.

As with any healing modality, you must have an understanding of your working tools before you can embark on treatment or healing. This knowledge increases, of course, as you form your own special relationship with the oils. As you experiment, you may find that some oils are not for you.

Others may have a euphoric effect. You are usually the best judge of what works—and this book has been written to provide you with the necessary knowledge to get started.

As a final cautionary note, it's important to take care when using citrus oils. Don't use them on the skin if you're going to be in direct sunlight, and be careful about how many drops you use in a bath. If you have sensitive skin, you may find that you don't want to use citrus oils while bathing.

With knowledge of what essential oils can do—and with intuition about how they can work for you personally—you can cultivate a nurturing and healing relationship with Mother Nature's healing aromas.

WAYS TO USE ESSENTIAL OILS

Since essential oils are highly concentrated, they must be diluted before they're used and not applied directly on the skin. You can use them in any of the following ways:

In a bath: Hopping into a warm bath at the end of a long day is one of life's most blissful moments. Add 5 to 8 drops of a blend of 3 oils before you climb into the bath. Agitate the water. Submerge your body to prepare yourself for the night ahead—whether you're staying at home for a quiet and relaxing time, going to a party, or spending a romantic evening with your lover. You can also use essential oils in the morning to invigorate and refresh you for the day ahead.

In a vaporizer: You can use a vaporizer at home or work to uplift or relax you. Vaporizers are used to fill the atmosphere with essential oils. Add 8 drops in total of your chosen combination of oils to the shallow dish filled with water at the top of the unit. Underneath, light a candle to heat the water and scent the air with healing vapors. You can choose oils to freshen the air, to assist with breathing, to aid concentration, or during a romantic interlude.

Massage: Massage is already a popular and highly respected way of loving and healing the body. Combine this with the use of essential oils, and you have a recipe for divine relaxation. A massage oil is a combination of essential oils added to a base oil—see Base Oils for more information. You can use massage oils to promote circulation, stimulate the release of toxins from the body, or uplift the senses—the list is endless. To every 10 milliliters (ml) of base oil, add 5 drops of essential oil (a 2:1 ratio).

Body rub: You can begin every day with energy and vitality by indulging in a two-minute body rub after your shower. When the body is warm, it absorbs oil quickly. Choose 3 essential oils to add to your base oil, and blend in a small bowl. Smooth the oil over the entire body to stimulate circulation and protect you during the day to come.

Inhalation: To help balance physical disorders and release emotions, you can inhale oils directly by adding 3 to 5 drops to a stainless steel or glass bowl filled with boiling water. Add the drops of essential oils to the water (agitate to release the vapors), place a towel over your head, and breathe deeply. For maximum benefit, keep your head over the bowl for 10 minutes. Remember to protect the sensitive eye area.

Compresses: Use a compress for facial skin care—it's useful for softening the skin and promoting cell regeneration—or for first aid to help relieve pain and swelling and reduce inflammation. Hot compresses are generally used to alleviate chronic pain, while cold compresses are ideal for acute pain and injury.

To make your compress, add 5 drops in total of your chosen 3 essential oils to a basin of hot or cold water. Fold a piece of gauze or a small towel, and soak it in the water. Squeeze out the excess water from the cloth, and apply it to the skin after the cloth has absorbed as much of the oil as possible from the surface of the water.

Spritzer: Ideal for summer, a spritzer hydrates and reenergizes the skin. This is a bottle with a nozzle that sprays water in a mistlike form. You can also use a spritzer to apply essential oils to wounds or burns. Using 90 ml of water, add 5 drops of a combination of 3 essential oils to a spritzer bottle.

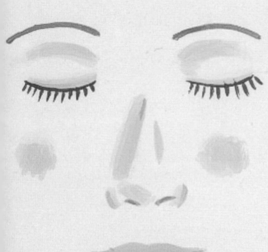

Lifestyle Tips

Essential oils have many applications for mind, body, and spirit. You can use them in all areas of your life to promote general well-being and to enhance the quality of any experience.

The Spirit

To fortify the spirit . . .

Black Pepper—Black Pepper is an oil for strength. With daily massage, it can dispel past anxieties and fortify a sense of confidence and adequacy. Combine with Lime and Cinnamon to encourage confidence in your own strength in the face of dire circumstances.

Dill—In ancient times, gladiators would rub their bodies with this pungently aromatic oil. It is a symbol of the healing spirit and the possibility of moving on. For those who like life to be balanced and controlled, and who feel knocked around when confronted with the natural highs and lows of life, Dill combined with Clary Sage and Geranium will establish an equilibrium. Dill assists you in staying true to your intentions.

Grieving—the loss of a loved one . . .

Cypress—Cypress in conjunction with Marjoram and Rose helps restore the body, bringing about new direction and comfort. Encouragement and assertion are sometimes needed when taking control and responsibility for one's life. This blend can support you when dealing with the loss of a loved one. For those experiencing regret, Cypress encourages a sense of straightforwardness and strengthens willpower. During the day, carry along a few drops of this blend on a tissue to give support during those moments when you need to step back and take it easy. Breathe in the oils, and give the situation some space. Allow your feelings to be expressed, and the oils to bring contentment and stillness to the moment.

Juniper +

Transformation . . .

Frankincense—Frankincense is a deeply spiritual oil that liberates you from the mundane. Blend with Basil and Everlasting (Everlasting is often referred to as Immortelle). This blend can direct you to your higher consciousness, a rare and humble wakefulness where discovery is possible.

Fears and nightmares . . .

Marjoram—Marjoram, Frankincense, and Orange as a blend can arrest the emotional charges that play on your subconscious and disturb your inner calm during sleep. This combination bathes you in the spirit of rejuvenation, as visions and thoughts that have disturbed your peace in the past are put to rest.

Healing old wounds . . .

Frankincense—Frankincense in conjunction with Myrrh and Juniper assists the closing of old wounds, both physical and emotional, especially those that continue to expel toxic waste from the body. This blend cleanses and purifies as it assists in facilitating change and transition.

Evoking passion . . .

Jasmine—Jasmine combined with Clary Sage and Rose permeates to the subconscious and helps release old beliefs that can restrain and repress you. This blend awakens passion and allows for the expression of your true desires.

Finding purpose and direction . . .

Lemon—Lemon, Myrrh, and Spikenard form a potent blend that grounds you as you step into the future, ensuring that your actions are in line with your intentions. These oils bring about clarity, esteem, and direction; they help you make the right decisions.

To strengthen and empower . . .

Melissa—Melissa can bring you to a place where human frailties are diminished. When blended with Geranium and Lavender, it strengthens those who feel oversensitive and find themselves detached and insecure.

Meditation . . .

Myrrh—Myrrh, used in a vaporizer during meditation, can purify and create an environment for the unfolding of inner wisdom and the acceptance of new teachings and awareness. Blend with Juniper and Sandalwood.

Tranquility . . .

Cedarwood—Cedarwood, combined with Rose and Palmarosa, nourishes the soul and restores inner calm. Find a quiet place, focus on your breathing, and deeply inhale the richness of this blend.

The Body

Morning kick-start . . .

Pine—Pine with Lemon and Cardamom stimulates circulation and mobilizes the body's cleansing system, providing a new level of energy and vitality to get you going. Body brushing with an aromatic wash in the shower eliminates toxins. Fill a small bottle with warm water, add 3 drops of your blend, sprinkle over your body, and brush in a circular motion.

Rosemary—Inhale Rosemary from a tissue prepared with a few drops of oil; this sharpens the mind and brings the senses alive so that they are fully engaged during the day. Use a body brush in the shower, and finish off with a Rosemary rinse to get the circulation going. A great way to wake up small children is to place a Rosemary tissue under their nose and gently shake their body all over to bring consciousness to their muscles.

Lemongrass—Lemongrass, with its potent aromatic influence, awakens the senses and assists in activating and energizing the body. Use a combination of Lemongrass, Cardamom, and Black Pepper in a morning blend to spice up your life!

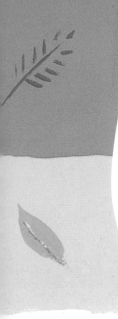

Regulating normal body functions . . .

Caraway—Caraway, in combination with Bay Laurel and Fennel, works particularly well when massaged on the abdominal area of the body to help with conditions such as diarrhea, flatulence, and constipation—or whenever the intestinal tract needs rebalancing. It assists in destroying the lingering flora that can produce dysfunction when eating rich and heavy foods such as red meat and cooked meats. It is excellent for an overworked intestinal tract when the body has been subjected to chronic overeating.

To move beyond fatigue . . .

Clary Sage—The symptoms of fatigue are felt both physically and emotionally, so when it's time to revive the sprit, use Clary Sage in combination with Thyme and Eucalyptus. Fill a glass spritzer bottle with water, add 2 drops of each essential oil, and shake to disperse the oils. When you're feeling tired, use the aromatic water to hydrate and revive.

Combating infection . . .

Ginger—Ginger is energizing and activating; it is a powerful tonic for the body, especially when combined with Thyme and Lime. This blend assists in counteracting the recurrence of viral and bacterial infections. Use in the winter months to protect the body.

Reshaping your body . . .

Fennel—Fennel, combined with Rosemary and Grapefruit, is the blend to use when you want to reshape and redefine your body's form. The sculpting of your new body begins with a daily massage, as the body tissue is mobilized and the cells respond to the touch and care you provide. Remember, the cells have their own intelligence and listen to the messages you give. Use 5 ml of Jojoba oil as a base, and add 3 drops of essential oil in total. Smooth the finest layer of oil over the entire body, daily, massaging it in as you go.

To relieve muscular aches and pains . . .

Everlasting—When muscles and joints are sprained or strained, this oil can be used as a compress or in baths to

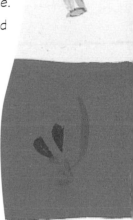

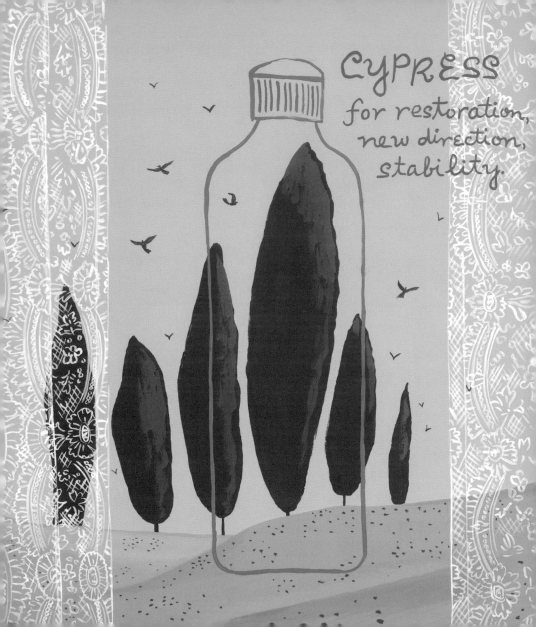

CYPRESS
for restoration,
new direction,
stability.

soothe and relax. Due to its ability to promote circulation, in conjunction with Juniper and Yarrow it makes an excellent body blend to help relieve discomfort and restriction.

Healing . . .

Clary Sage—Use during times of convalescence when you're feeling impatient. When combined with Lavender and Patchouli, it tends to reinstate ease and comfort, while healing and repairing scar tissue.

Skin care . . .

Glowing skin is a true reflection of your inner well-being. Ensure that your complexion radiates vitality by adding a blend of Palmarosa, Geranium, and Neroli to a base of Jojoba, a fluid wax, to use as your daily moisturizer.

Sandalwood—Sandalwood with Rose and Lavender is the perfect blend to use on a daily basis to regenerate and prevent dryness and dehydration. Your skin-care program of today will determine the quality of your skin tomorrow. A few drops in a compress application, or added to Jojoba, moisturizes and nourishes the skin.

Sage—Sage, Cypress, and Lemon control excess oil in the skin. When blended into Jojoba and massaged into the skin, the oils work to deeply cleanse and rebalance the skin. This blend is far more effective than using an astringent, which only makes the oil glands work double time.

Orange—When the skin takes on an orange-peel appearance with dirty pores, Orange clears out the toxins and decongests the skin. Combined with Sage and Cypress, this oil encourages the skin to look cleaner, fresher, and more hydrated. It is an excellent skin tonic.

Hair treatments . . .

Add your chosen essential oils to a bottle of shampoo or water to pour through your hair as a final rinse. Use Tea Tree with Cedarwood and Rosemary for dandruff, a blend of Chamomile and Lemon for fair hair, or Sandalwood for adding luster to dark hair.

For Travel

Flying . . .

Caraway—Caraway is very good for those who travel frequently, as well as those who are fearful of heights, as it is said to diminish vertigo.

In combination with Frankincense and Palmarosa, it allays fears and acts as an effective skin regenerator. This is particularly helpful when you're traveling. Add 2 drops of each essential oil to a glass spritzer bottle filled with water, and spritz your face regularly before and during the flight.

Ginger—With its warming, digestive function and balancing effect, Ginger is an excellent travel companion for those who suffer from travel sickness. In conjunction with Orange and Roman Chamomile, it should be massaged onto the abdominal area, especially if eating and sitting for long periods. It acts as a preventive measure. If nausea persists, inhale Peppermint.

First aid . . .

Cypress—The cooling effect of Cypress works effectively with German Chamomile and Tea Tree on inflamed skin conditions, and is especially effective where there is discharge around a wound.

Tea Tree—This antiseptic oil is a favorite choice for first aid—you can put a few drops onto a bandage and place it over the skin, or place it directly onto an insect bite or wound.

Lavender—Lavender is used to heal and repair injury to the skin, stemming from sunburn or burns from heating devices or boiling water.

It prevents scarring and promotes regeneration. Make a poultice using honey, and apply it to the skin, or simply add a few drops to water as a wash. Lavender can be applied neat on small areas; use only 1 drop.

Oregano—Oregano is a potent tonic; it's useful as a preventive oil when venturing into harsh environments, or when there is uncertainty about sanitary conditions. Blend with Tea Tree and Eucalyptus to cleanse your environment and contact surfaces.

In the Home

For dining . . .

Caraway—Place a few drops of Caraway along with Ginger and Lime in your vaporizer before the guests arrive. This will create a calm atmosphere ready for sumptuous dining. These stimulating oils will get the digestive juices flowing.

In the family room . . .

In the cold of winter, dispense several drops of Pine and Sandalwood onto the logs of the open fire. The relaxing qualities of Sandalwood with

Smooth

the refreshing aroma of Pine will enhance your quality time with friends and family.

Lavender—A few drops of Lavender, along with Orange and Palmarosa in your vaporizer, can stir your senses. As you let go of the troubles of the day, this comforting ambience restores and calms.

In the bedroom . . .

Marjoram—Marjoram creates a delightful environment for slumber, a haven that will function like a cocoon for you. The following blend prepared in the vaporizer diffuses to create an ambience in which you can surrender your mind, body, and emotions. Add Orange, Lavender, and Marjoram to your vaporizer—use a total of 8 drops—and light it at least half an hour before retiring.

Neroli—For a touch of elegance and grace, spray Neroli between the sheets of your bed. Simply add 5 drops to a spritzer bottle filled with water, and spray a light mist over the linens. This sweet aromatic, blended with Lavender and Cardamom, will create a sense of indulgence as you climb into bed.

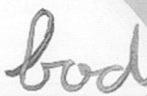

In the bathroom . . .

Spikenard–Spikenard, together with Rosewood and Bergamot, helps you relax and unwind at the end of a busy day. The troubles of the day are surrendered as the combination of warm water and aromatic bliss nurtures your body and mind.

Peppermint–One drop of Peppermint and Tea Tree added to a cup of water can be used as a mouthwash before retiring.

In Relationships

For romance . . .

Ylang Ylang–Create a blend that speaks to you, which will evoke the senses and arouse the body. Combine Ylang Ylang with Rose for the heart, and Mandarin for spontaneity and joy. As you smooth the blend over your body, your body heat will act as the diffuser, sending the oils into the air and subtly seducing your lover.

Creating the mood . . .

Candlelight sets the perfect environment for romance. The subtlety of the light, coupled with 1 drop of your favorite oil added to the candle, will evoke the senses. Try Patchouli, Jasmine, or Mandarin.

For an aromatic signature, dispense several drops of your favorite oil onto a piece of blotting paper or a cotton ball, and tuck it inside a lidded box with your cards or paper. The fragrance will permeate through the paper. To rekindle the message sent, wear the blend at any time.

Lavender—Lavender is an excellent oil to use for setting a serene mood in a home environment when clear communication is needed. For those who feel vulnerable, oversensitive, and inhibited by emotions, Lavender reassures and allows communication to flow more easily.

Petitgrain—Petitgrain brings inner vision and strength, and helps stabilize the emotions. When blended with Ylang Ylang and Sandalwood in your vaporizer, you have the perfect combination for expressing yourself confidently while creating a forum for open communication.

At the Gym

Sage—Smelly shoes and sweaty feet can be refreshed with Sage, Lime, and Cypress. Spritz the feet by adding 3 drops of each oil to a small spritzer bottle filled with water.

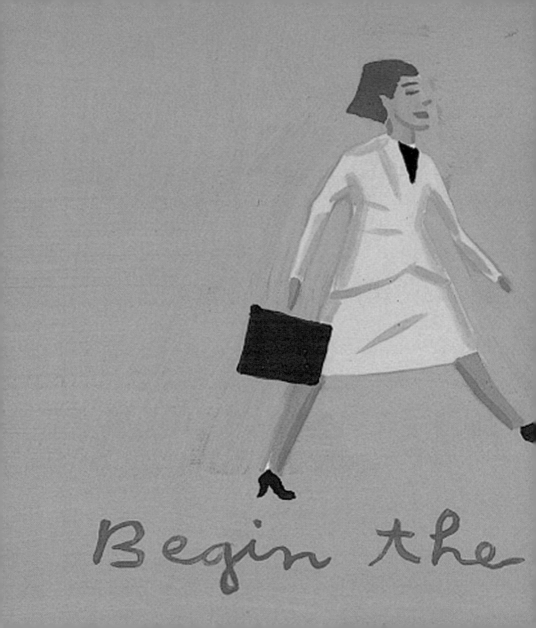

Begin the

Eucalyptus–Eucalyptus oxygenates your body quickly, and revives your focus. Blend with Black Pepper and Lemongrass in Jojoba for endurance and performance. Rub your body down with the oils before and after training.

At the Office

Fennel–Use Fennel for new possibilities in board meetings. Combine with Grapefruit for spontaneity and Basil for focus. Fennel and Basil make an excellent blend when you want to promote communication and implement new ideas.

For learning and concentration . . .

Bay–Bay, with Rosemary and Lime, reactivates the mind, expands awareness, and opens up new learning opportunities.

Pine–Pine, with Eucalyptus and Hyssop, improves concentration as it oxygenates the body. Stimulating alertness, these oils work especially well in air-conditioned environments that feel stuffy and congested.

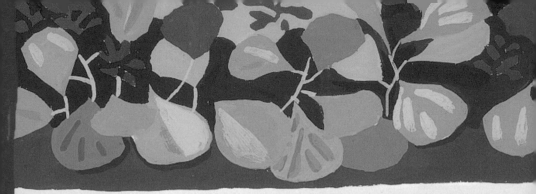

Peppermint—Peppermint is useful when preparing for study, especially after lunch when midafternoon lethargy can kick in. Instead of coffee or a chocolate bar, fill your desk vaporizer with this stimulating digestive aid that sharpens the senses, engages the mind, and helps you "digest" information. Blend with Lime and Black Pepper.

Lemon—Use Lemon for clear communication. Blend with Tea Tree to use as a disinfectant. A couple of drops wiped over the mouthpiece of the telephone can protect you from viruses and bacteria.

Lavender—A drop of Lavender placed on the pulse points allays frustrations and calms the mind. When the going gets tough and it all seems like a little too much, take yourself into nature by inhaling Lavender.

Grapefruit—Grapefruit is particularly valuable when you're feeling tense and overburdened, with too much to do. It helps stimulate spontaneity and creativity, and in combination with Bay and Rosemary, it makes an excellent blend for high performance in professional environments. Fill a cup with very hot water, dispense your drops into the cup, and inhale deeply.

For Women

Geranium—Geranium nourishes the feminine qualities and instills a sense of assuredness and stability. Geranium quells anxiety and allows for greater intimacy to be expressed in relationships. Used in a bath with Lavender and Cedarwood, it activates balance, stability, and comfort. This blend has regenerating qualities and addresses discontent and oversensitivity.

During menopause . . .

Clary Sage—With maturity, you move to an inner knowing and wisdom. This oil helps transform your knowledge into wisdom, and turn everyday tasks into mindful practices. Clary Sage is known to be the most euphoric of all essential oils. When self-doubt undermines your inner knowing, choose this oil to reconnect with your wisdom. This oil brings about comfort in times of confrontation and grief.

Clary Sage helps release fear and opens up the possibility for insight that is available to women during menopause. Combine with Geranium and Frankincense for best results.

Jasmine—Jasmine brings balance to hormonal changes or disruptions; and regularity during times of upheaval such as adolescence, menopause, menstruation, and postoperative care. When combined with Lavender and Geranium, it inspires balance, and provides you with the opportunity to get back in touch with your inner source of creativity.

Menstruation . . .

Cypress—Cypress helps balance the flow of blood and energy in the entire reproductive area. Use in conjunction with Basil and Roman Chamomile as a tonic to strengthen and balance the energy and vitality of your inner strength.

For Men

Bergamot—Bergamot with Lavender can be used as an aftershave blend, or for use on sensitive skin. Add to a cup of water along with Cedarwood and Tea Tree for use as an aftershave splash. Men with sensitive skin can add a combination of Lavender, Bergamot, and Sandalwood oils to a massage base oil.

Rosemary—Rosemary added to Cedarwood and Juniper oils stimulates hair growth. Add to a base oil, and massage into your hair and scalp.

For Children

Sandalwood–Sandalwood, Cypress, and Lemon help protect and stabilize when a young one feels sensitive and emotionally vulnerable. A few drops on a cotton ball placed inside their pillow does the trick.

Roman Chamomile–Roman Chamomile and Lavender soothe an aching tummy, and also quell the emotions. Dispense 3 drops of each oil into a warm bath, or on a compress cloth.

Let your children choose their own favorite oils. They will develop their intuition when they are left to be guided by their sense of smell. Some favorites are: Orange, Lavender, Chamomile, Sandalwood, Geranium, and Mandarin.

Base Oils

For a massage or body rub blend, add essential oils to one of the following base oils. Remember to keep your base oil blends in glass containers. Also, vegetable oils will become rancid after a while, so use them within six to eight months. Macadamia and Jojoba oils can last for several years.

Jojoba—Jojoba oil is high in protein and minerals, and is a natural wax fluid. This oil rejuvenates and nourishes skin and hair.

Peach Kernel—Peach Kernel oil is high in vitamin A and helps promote a rosy complexion. As a massage oil base, it moisturizes and softens the skin.

Olive—Olive oil is rich in proteins and vitamins and brings warmth to the body as a massage base oil. It is particularly beneficial as a body rub during winter.

Sweet Almond—Sweet Almond oil is light, and perfect for massage. Place a few drops on your body, and your hands will glide effortlessly over your skin for a soothing massage.

Wheat Germ—Wheat Germ oil is high in vitamin E; as such, it is great for the skin, especially skin that's scarred. As an antioxidant, Wheat Germ also extends the life span of your essential oils by preventing oxidation.

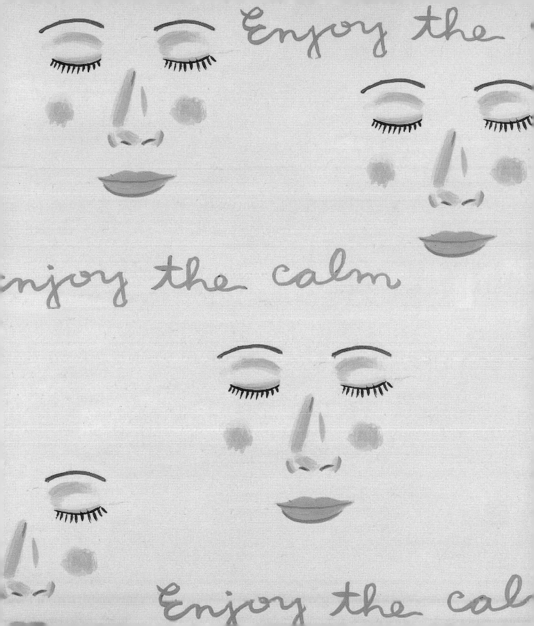

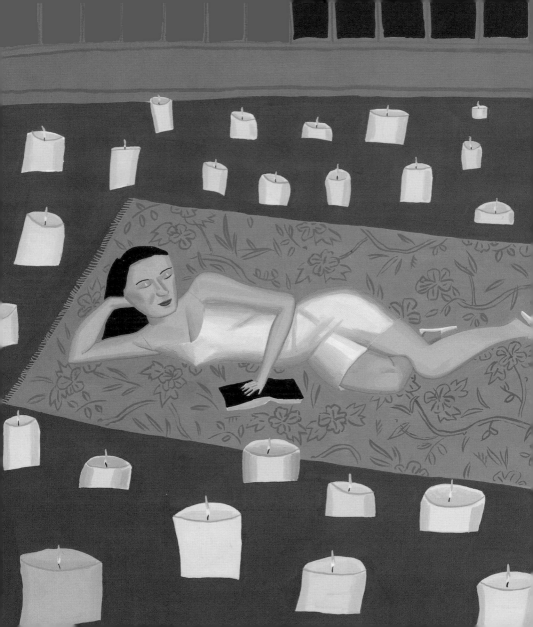

A—Z of Essential Oils

BASIL (ocimum basilicum)

Basil originated in Asia and the Pacific Islands. This flowering plant grows to a height of about six inches. The oil is extracted from the green leaves of the herb.

Basil has commonly been used in India for its sacred qualities. It is said that Lords Krishna and Vishnu endowed themselves with it for protection. Basil has traditionally been taken as a part of religious and spiritual ceremonies to enhance inspiration.

As a potent aromatic rub, Basil can be used to purify. Excellent on muscle spasms of the respiratory tract and chest area, it is especially helpful in wintertime for stimulating your sense of smell when colds and congestion ravage the body. Leaf oils such as Basil are good respiratory aids that are used to expand the chest.

Basil is most effective in helping to clarify and focus thoughts; it is a great aid in decision-making. It activates the brain when the mind is flagging and needs to be revived. In times of doubt and confusion, applying Basil to the head brings clarity and helps you refocus on the task at hand.

When sitting down to concentrate or study, Basil helps align concentration and intention.

In ancient times, Basil was used to purge the body of fever, making it a great companion to Eucalyptus oil. As a preventive measure and for self-healing, it can be massaged onto the chest in combination with other oils for bronchitis, emphysema, and muscular spasms. It is a stimulating tonic for congested skin.

Applied to joint areas where rheumatoid arthritis is producing discomfort, it alleviates pain. Its cooling qualities dissipate the heat and irritability associated with rheumatic pain.

Basil is a great tonic for the nervous system, especially when feeling vulnerable or fragile. Basil tends to sharpen the senses, and it can bring about a state of alert wakefulness, especially when feeling overwhelmed. This oil acts as a wonderful tonic for those with a nervous disposition.

During the day's activities, use Basil as a pick-me-up.

IT ADDRESSES: Apprehension, confusion, nervous exhaustion, lethargy, depression, loss of memory, feeling overwhelmed, irregular periods, congested skin, spasmodic coughing, headaches, migraines, indigestion, muscle spasms, insect bites, gout.

IT HELPS PROMOTE: Clear thinking, mobility, energy, alertness, good decision-making, improved digestion, restoration of the nervous system, menstrual rhythm.

SAFETY INFORMATION: Do not use during pregnancy, as it stimulates menstruation.

BAY (Pimenta acris)

Don't confuse Bay with Bay Laurel (see below). Bay is a small evergreen tree growing wild in the West Indies and Venezuela. The essential oil is extracted from the bay leaf.

Traditionally, Bay has been used for both its culinary and medicinal qualities. As a hair tonic, it helps stimulate hair growth and adds luster. With its warm and spicy aroma, it uplifts despondent moods.

Bay is excellent as an analgesic, carrying with it antiseptic qualities. It has a stimulating effect as an expectorant on the chest and lungs. Use for flus, coughs, colds, bronchitis, and pneumonia.

Bay is known for its ability to release and relieve muscle

spasms and strains, thus making it an excellent liniment for poor circulation or for use after training. It also alleviates cramps, flatulence, and indigestion. For any condition associated with stagnation or lack of mobility, apply topically to the body in a massage blend.

As it activates the body and the senses, it is also effective in treating impotency and emotional frigidity. It has a mobilizing effect, helping you move toward a more open expression of sexuality. As a resource for those working in the creative arts, it promotes the flow of creativity.

Bay is an excellent oil to use when energy is lacking, particularly when chronic nervous tension and exhaustion are present. It brings ease and warmth to the body and the emotions, and energizes when stamina is needed. It is excellent for dejected moods, encouraging you to move forward with zest.

It ADDRESSES: Hair loss, pneumonia, colds, coughs, flus, sinusitis, muscle spasms, poor circulation, flatulence, lack of stamina, exhaustion, nervous tension.

It HELPS PROMOTE: Strength, creativity, stamina, energy, warmth, a general sense of well-being, stimulation of the body and senses, the fighting off of infections, protection of the body.

SAFETY INFORMATION: Do not use on mucous membranes or highly sensitive skin.

BAY LAUREL (Laurus nobilis)

The Bay Laurel (Laurus) is a sturdy evergreen tree found native in Southern Europe, where the essential oil is extracted from the leaf of the plant. The Romans and Egyptians used it widely in ancient times as a symbol of wisdom, protection, and peace. The Latin name for this oil means "to praise"; hence, the presentation of laurel wreaths to victors at the Olympic games.

Bay Laurel can be used for respiratory disorders, especially where there is infection and congestion. With the help of Eucalyptus and Cedarwood, it is excellent for opening up and decongesting the lungs.

This oil is an active digestive aid and assists in dispelling gas from the intestinal tract while also acting as a tonic for indigestion. Use in a blend with Caraway and Fennel. In combination with Grapefruit, this oil makes a great tonic for the liver and promotes the flow of digestive juices.

Bay Laurel is good in the bath and in a massage blend for relieving muscular aches, pains, and sprains, especially in combination with Juniper and Lavender. Use in combination with Eucalyptus and Lemongrass after exercise.

Use Bay Laurel to promote activity when feeling cold during the winter months—when used with Eucalyptus, it is excellent for reducing fever.

In combination with Basil and Roman Chamomile, Bay Laurel is particularly effective for irregular and scanty menstruation. It helps strengthen and stimulate the immune system, especially when the body is recovering from illness. During convalescence, it acts as a pick-me-up.

As a remedy for the hair and scalp, Bay Laurel stimulates growth and helps clear up dandruff.

Stimulating to the mind, Bay Laurel can be used when feeling overwhelmed, or when you want to say the right thing at the right time. A great time to use this oil is during exams or when going for a job interview—anytime that anxiety, fear, and doubt can override clarity and purpose.

Bay Laurel is an antidepressant and is excellent for those who tend to be morbid or pessimistic. It stimulates confidence, inspiration, and self-esteem.

IT ADDRESSES: Doubt, fear, low self-esteem, pessimism, congestion, coughs, colds, fevers, muscular aches and pains, muscle stiffness, irregular and painful menstruation, liver congestion, slow digestion, colic.

IT HELPS PROMOTE: Clear thinking, inspiration, self-esteem, insight, intuition, good digestion and liver function, expectorant action in the lungs, energy, confidence.

SAFETY INFORMATION: Do not use undiluted on the skin, since it may irritate. Do not use on mucous membranes. Do not use during pregnancy.

BERGAMOT (Citrus bergamia)

This small citrus tree, native to tropical Asia, is widely cultivated in Calabria in Southern Italy, and is also grown on the Ivory Coast of Africa. The fruit is much like a small orange in appearance and ripens to a green-yellow color.

Tradition has it that Bergamot was named after the Italian city of the same name in Lombardy, where the oil was first extracted. For many years since, it has been used in Italian folk medicine to treat fever, and much like Basil, it has been used in India for the prevention and cure of malaria. It has a sweet, fruity smell with a slightly spicy undertone. It is well known for its applications to physical and emotional states of imbalance.

In Italian folklore, Bergamot appeared as an antiseptic, and in Napoleonic times, it was especially favored as a perfume and eau de toilette. Bergamot is an excellent oil to use for nervous indigestion and overeating caused by a need to feed restless energy in the body.

With anti-infectious and antiseptic qualities, it can be used as a wash over the body for wounds, and is particularly beneficial against parasitic infections. Used with Tea Tree and Sandalwood, it treats throat infections.

In conjunction with Sage, Bergamot is excellent as a deodorant and expectorant for sweaty bodies. On the skin, it has the capacity to regenerate, especially when the skin's condition is linked to chronic stress conditions, such as with dermatitis, psoriasis, and eczema. Bergamot helps balance emotional states, and also settles disharmony of the skin.

Bergamot assists in balancing nervous conditions associated with eating disorders such as anorexia nervosa, and also quells overeating and abdominal distension and indigestion. It is especially useful when massaged over the digestive tract and the abdomen in conjunction with other digestive oils such as Cardamom and Fennel. The spicy flavors blend delightfully with the citrus.

Use Bergamot to help dissipate mild anxiety attacks, especially when confronted with feelings of fear or butterflies. This oil addresses the immediacy of the challenge when faced with the unexpected.

Bergamot's light and refreshing aroma diffuses readily into any environment, and impacts profoundly on the nervous system, settling anxiety.

Bergamot's gentle, relaxing effect uplifts the senses, and energetically, it has the ability to promote harmony and restore a sense of vitality throughout the body and mind.

Bergamot helps establish a sense of lighthearted-ness, thus having a profound effect on those who dwell in the past and tend to procrastinate. It helps dissipate tension and frustration, and it loosens past residues. This oil helps release feelings that have been suppressed, which have led to depression or anxiety. Relax and let go with Bergamot.

IT ADDRESSES: Wounds, infections in the body, ulcers, indigestion, dermatitis, psoriasis, excessive perspiration, genito-urinary infections, poor appetite, nervous butterflies, acute nervous disorders, sadness, depression, despondency.

IT HELPS PROMOTE: Motivation, fulfillment, contentment, clear skin, good digestion, balance in the genito-urinary system, regeneration of the skin, uplifting of the mind, calmness, a sense of balance, ease.

SAFETY INFORMATION: Phototoxic; do not use in the presence of sunlight or UV light. It may also be irritating to extremely sensitive skin.

GERANIUM for harmony, balance, security, comfort, regularity in menstrual cycle.

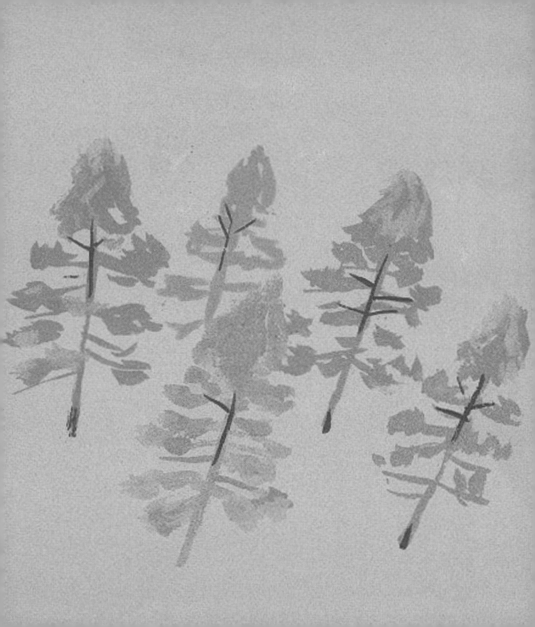

BIRCH (Betula lenta)

Birch oil is taken from the bark and twigs of the tree. It is first soaked in water to free the essential oil before distillation.

Because of its strength and height, the Birch tree has traditionally been used for its protective qualities and to ward off evil spirits. From time immemorial, it has been used to make medicinal wines and as a tea for diuretic purposes. It has impressive astringent qualities, and is also an excellent oil to use in skin tonics and body liniments.

As an antispasmodic oil, in conjunction with Basil, it addresses disorders of the respiratory and pulmonary tracts. It is an antirheumatic oil and can be used in a massage blend with Eucalyptus and Juniper to apply to arthritic and rheumatic conditions. It has a disinfectant quality, and is often used as a liver tonic to release toxic buildup in the body. Birch stimulates the lymphatic system and can be used as a preventive measure against infections.

Birch is particularly good for strengthening bones and joints; it restores and heals.

Birch helps treat scalp conditions such as dandruff and flaking skin. As an antiseptic, it has a purifying and cleansing effect on the scalp. It is excellent to use as a compress in conjunction with Sage for congested skin and acne conditions.

Used as an aid to reshape the body, Birch diminishes the buildup

of toxins and increases the flow of urine—
thereby assisting with water retention, cellulite, and obesity.
With its capacity to stimulate the liver, it makes a great blend with
Grapefruit and Rosemary to control obesity and weight loss.

Birch has an invigorating effect on the mind, so when combined with Basil, it is great for alleviating headaches and mental strain when dealing with facts, figures, and statistics. Birch and Basil are particularly effective in relieving the overburden of too much left-brain activity.

Given its height and strength, on a psychological level, Birch helps elevate self-worth, while at the same time encouraging generosity. It promotes openness (a trait inherent in its branches—which have a tendency to open to the sky). It can also invigorate the mind and allow for a new perspective, since it diminishes worry.

> **IT ADDRESSES:** Worry, obesity, a sluggish lymphatic system, dandruff, congested skin, immobility due to stiff joints, infections, rheumatic complaints, water retention, cellulite.

> **IT HELPS PROMOTE:** Strength, self-worth, openness, weight reduction, body tone, strength in joints, healthy hair, invigoration of body and mind, cleansing of the body, restoration of the skin.

> **SAFETY INFORMATION:** Avoid on sensitive or damaged skin. Do not use during pregnancy.

BLACK PEPPER (Piper nigrum)

The essential oil of Black Pepper is extracted from the peppercorns, known as the fruit of the plant. It is widely grown in India, Indonesia, and Madagascar, where it is cultivated for both its culinary and medicinal qualities.

Its sharp and spicy aroma activates and excites the body. It is a revered spice in India and has always been used for urinary tract and liver complaints. It is mostly associated with conditions suffered in tropical countries—cholera and dysentery—during times when medicines are difficult to obtain.

Black Pepper warms up the body in preparation for a tough cardiovascular workout by helping to increase circulation and the lymphatic flow. It is excellent for muscle aches and pains when added to a warm bath, and it is good for toning muscles—especially in those who have been convalescing or bedridden for some time. Also, use for conditions where energy and vitality are required in the muscular system, such as temporary paralysis, stiffness of joints, or body strains and pains.

Black Pepper is a great chest rub for chronic bronchitis because it alleviates and removes congestion in the respiratory system. During the winter months, when you're feeling chilled, use it to bring warmth to the joints, and to promote circulatory flow to the extremities of the body—your feet and hands.

Black Pepper can be used with Juniper to assist the flow of blood where bruising and wounds have occurred on the body. It is excellent as a preventive measure against infections, colds and coughs, flus and viruses, tonsillitis, and laryngitis.

Black Pepper oil is one of the most popular ones for energizing and stimulating the body. It is a great tonic for nervous conditions, and it helps you maintain energy levels when the going gets tough—especially when the mind has been overworked, and endurance is required by the body.

When you are confronted with rapid change, Black Pepper is an excellent oil for disorientation and fatigue, and it is especially effective for decision-making when faced with adversity. When others are behaving irrationally around you, Black Pepper can keep you focused and on track, helping you resist the temptation to shut down during challenging circumstances.

Black Pepper is excellent for enhancing enthusiasm and providing the vitality and energy required to get the job done; it releases any tendency to be apathetic, bringing about a sense of certainty and direction.

Black Pepper fortifies the spirit—it is the oil to use to spice up your life.

IT ADDRESSES: Lethargy, boredom, physical and mental fatigue, irrational behavior, bronchitis, colds, winter chills, poor circulation, a slow metabolism, muscular aches and pains, paralysis, bruising, joint stiffness.

IT HELPS PROMOTE: Warmth, stimulation, enthusiasm, energy and vitality to body and mind, mobility, circulatory flow, stimulation of the lymphatic system, muscle tone, good respiratory function, decongestion.

SAFETY INFORMATION: Do not use on open or inflamed skin. Can be an irritant to highly sensitive skin. Not to be used in large doses.

BORNEOL (Dryobalanops aromatica)

With its towering height and thick trunk, this tree is majestic. The oil is found in the crevices of the bark of the tree just below the surface, and is known as liquid camphor.

During the Dark Ages, when herbal law reigned as the medicine of the day, Borneol was used as a powerful antidote and preventive measure against the Plague and other severe infectious diseases. Known to the ancient Chinese for its pungent aromas and its preserving qualities, Borneol was used in embalming.

With its anti-infectious capacities, Borneol can be used during the winter months to stimulate the immune system to fight colds, fevers, and flus. It is also helpful to use when feeling debilitated due to poor circulation, or resisting remnants of infections in the body. It is an excellent oil for recovery.

Borneol is an analgesic, easing pain and desensitizing local areas when applied to strains and sprains. It relieves tension in the neck and shoulders. It helps ease discomfort of the physical body and allows you to rebuild, restore, and move on. In conjunction with

Juniper and Lavender, it can be used on the skin for bruises. It also acts as an insect repellent.

A stimulant to the adrenals to mobilize the body, Borneol is also said to have a stimulating effect on the sexual senses of the body, encouraging responsiveness.

For the mind and emotions, Borneol is an excellent oil for assisting with nervous strain, or when nervous exhaustion is apparent in relation to heavy demands that result in stress. When you're feeling burdened by thoughts and worries, there is a depletion of energy. With regular use of this oil, you'll feel encouraged to take risks as your energy builds.

IT ADDRESSES: Muscle stiffness and pain, bruising, physical tension, stress, nervous strain, neuralgia, debilitation, poor circulation, long-term infections.

IT HELPS PROMOTE: Recovery, restoration, energy, courage, momentum, healing, stimulation of the immune system, healing throughout the body, physical and emotional support.

SAFETY INFORMATION: Do not use during pregnancy, or with babies and young children under the age of five. It can be an irritant in high concentrations.

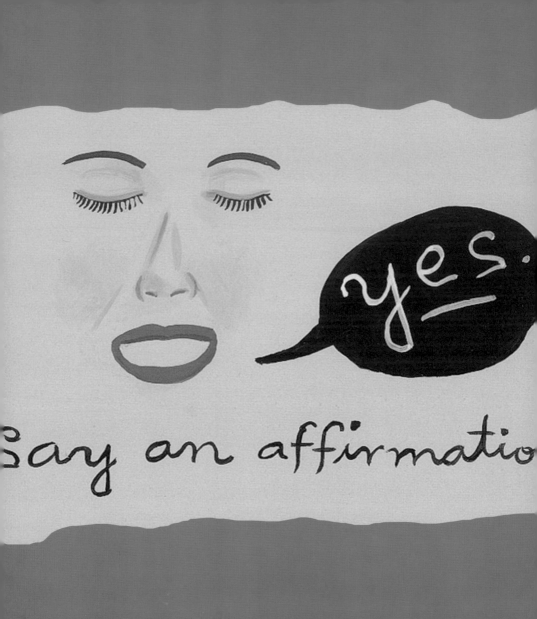

CAJEPUT (melaleuca cajeputi)

This tree of the melaleuca family is found growing wild throughout Asian and Australian environments. As a tall and powerful evergreen, the message it brings to the earth is one of endurance, as it does not surrender its leaves to the autumn and winter months. The essential oil is extracted from the leaf of the tree.

As an anti-infectious and congestion-fighting oil, it decongests the chest and acts as a potent expectorant for asthma, bronchitis, coughs, or when dealing with any disorders of the respiratory tract.

Cajeput is an overall tonic for the body, bringing a sensation of warmth and vitality to the whole circulatory system. It energizes the pulmonary system and strengthens varicose veins and hemorrhoids. It is used to address disorders of the circulatory system and as a remedy for the urinary tract.

For areas in the body where mobility or circulation is lacking—due to conditions such as arthritis, sprains, strains, or sports injuries—Cajeput is fantastic, as it helps alleviate muscular aches and pains. It also stimulates the immune system during the winter months and acts as a preventive measure against colds, flus, and viral infections.

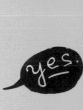

Cajeput is used for its antiseptic qualities, and is excellent as a gargle for sore throats and tonsillitis.

Cajeput oil activates and clears the head. As a stimulant, it is effective against procrastination when your mind feels congested. It brings energy and vitality to decision-making. Use this oil when you want to mobilize and bring new direction or new circumstances to your life, or when you need time out to rethink a decision.

IT ADDRESSES: Pulmonary, respiratory, and circulatory disorders; hemorrhoids; arthritis; sprains; infections; hardened conditions in the body; lack of vitality; congested thinking; being stuck in the past.

IT HELPS PROMOTE: A healthy immune system, good circulation, energy and vitality, strengthening of natural body functions, the fighting of bacteria, decongestion.

SAFETY INFORMATION: May irritate mucous membranes. Do not use during pregnancy. Do not use on inflamed conditions or highly sensitized skin.

CAMPHOR (Cinnamonum camphora)

This hardy evergreen tree, tall and adorned with white and red berries, has lived long in Eastern environments. While its life span can extend to 1,000 years, oil is not extracted from the tree until it is at least 50 years old. The essential oil is found in every part of the tree and takes many years to reach maturity. Of the three types of Camphor, the most preferable for aromatherapy is White Camphor, which doesn't contain saffron and is relatively nontoxic.

Historically, Eastern civilizations have used the plant for ceremonial purposes—at the end of battles, heroes would often be adorned with Camphor leaves as their crowning glory. Camphor boxes were used to preserve fabrics, and the oil is known for its preserving and protecting qualities.

Camphor is widely considered a stimulating oil, and activates areas where there is stiffness and restriction. As such, it's helpful for relieving arthritis, muscular aches, sprains and strains, and also rheumatism. It is particularly useful in chronic conditions where there has been pain or contusions. For winter chills, apply topically in a massage blend to best utilize its warming and activating properties.

Camphor oil's anti-inflammatory properties help it act as a cleansing agent for abscesses, wounds, and sores.

Camphor has a potent aroma, so it is effective for use when feeling faint or generally debilitated. As a stimulating oil, it brings balance to those who have been in a depressed or nervous state. It is an arousing oil and can help bring you out of a slump. It is especially beneficial during convalescence.

Whether you have issues to confront or an inability to focus mentally, Camphor can reactivate you and bring you back in line.

When there is too much mental activity at work and this interferes with your capacity to take up the challenge of life, Camphor restores strength of mind and initiative.

IT ADDRESSES: Debilitation, long-term physical conditions, muscle stiffness, immobility due to arthritis, winter chills, muscle weakness, depression, infections, inflammation.

IT HELPS PROMOTE: Mobility, stimulation, warmth, inner strength, initiative, focus, energy, preservation of the nervous system, cleansing of wound sites.

SAFETY INFORMATION: Yellow Camphor is toxic and is considered carcinogenic; it should never be used in therapy, either internally or externally.

White Camphor is relatively nontoxic and can be safely used topically. Do not use during pregnancy or on babies.

CARAWAY (Carum carvi)

This herb, with its feathery leaves and small flowers, bears its fruit in autumn. The essential oil is extracted from the ripe fruit or seeds, which are crushed before distillation. The plant is native to Europe, Siberia, and North Africa. While it is most widely cultivated for its culinary applications, it is commonly used in healing.

In ancient times, Caraway was used by the Romans to assist with digestion and flatulence. In India, it has a reputation for sweetening the breath and is always served after meals. With its warm, spicy, and stimu-lating attributes, Caraway has the capacity to promote circulation. It is an oil for vitality and energy, stimulating digestion and activating thought. In medieval times, it was used as a love potion. Today, we can use this oil to encourage commitment in love.

On a physical level, Caraway oil helps the small and large intestines to process food. It assists with the muscular functions of this area, stimulating peristaltic action. In combination with Fennel and Peppermint, it is excellent for digestion. To relax the abdomen and stimulate colon action, blend Caraway with Marjoram.

This is an oil that can be used to mobilize fat in the body. Its digestive actions and warming qualities help to break down stagnant areas caused by fat deposits in the body.

During unstable emotional times, when demands are made on you, or when you're feeling particularly fearful, it helps to bring about a sense of composure, thus encouraging the confidence and reassurance to move on. Caraway promotes commitment and stability when feeling doubt.

Caraway is extracted from the seeds of the plant; therefore, it embodies the essence of renewal—giving birth to newness and creativity. It also has a reputation for regenerating an old relationship or a future goal.

Caraway increases milk flow in nursing mothers, just as Fennel does, and is a general tonic for the immune system. In conjunction with Juniper and Lavender, it is an excellent remedy for bruises and infected wound sites.

Caraway is a skin regenerator, helps treat cellulite, and acts as a stimulant to the lymphatic system. In ancient times, it was used to bring color to pale complexions.

As a seed oil, Caraway acts as a general nerve tonic, tends to get you going, eases mental strain, replenishes loss of energy, and aids liver and gall bladder functions.

IT ADDRESSES: Instability, uncertainty, being stuck in the past, wound infections, a sluggish lymphatic system, excess body fat, cellulite, slow digestion.

IT HELPS PROMOTE: Body sculpting, good digestion, a healthy immune system, milk flow in nursing mothers, skin replenishment, a healthy complexion, proper gall bladder function.

SAFETY INFORMATION: Do not use during pregnancy, or with babies and young children under age eight.

CARDAMOM (Elettaria cardamomum)

The long, silky, blade-shaped leaves of this herb attest to its ability to instill a sense of motivation and enthusiasm in people. It is extracted from the seeds of the plant, and as a spice oil, blends well with other spice and citrus oils. It has traditionally been used in India, Europe, and China for its medicinal applications. Chewing Cardamom seeds is said to give you sweetness of breath.

Cardamom is excellent for sciatica associated with muscular spasms, pertaining to both the chest and abdominal area. It is particularly beneficial when deficiencies are evident in the body, and as a result, the body is tired and lethargic.

As a stimulant, Cardamon acts as an expectorant, ridding the body of inflammation in the chest cavity. It also helps relieve coughs, colds, and bronchitis. It is a great tonic to warm the body when winter chills persist.

Nervous conditions and digestive disorders such as vomiting, dyspepsia, or diarrhea can benefit from a Cardamom massage blend to restore vitality and energy to the body.

Use Cardamom for PMS symptoms to balance irregular or absent menstruation.

Cardamom helps dispel worry and concern, establishing inner contentment in those who feel burdened with responsibility. It can be considered an aphrodisiac because it unleashes creativity and an appetite for life. Warming, uplifting, and invigorating, it is an oil for inspiring opportunity, generosity, and for arousing sensuality.

Cardamom reminds you of all of the possibilities in life; you set aside your worries and concerns to find that as one door closes, another one opens. Cardamom helps you move forward with inner resolve and stability. It can restore your appetite for life.

IT ADDRESSES: Lethargy, sore and tired muscles, bad breath, digestive disorders, dyspepsia, diarrhea, low energy, tension in the body and mind, winter chills, despondency.

It helps promote: Endurance, mobility, momentum, fulfillment, stimulation, contentment, a healthy appetite, generosity, inner warmth.

Safety information: Do not use during pregnancy. It's a possible irritant on sensitive or allergic skin types.

CARROT SEED (Daucus carota)

This seed oil is extracted from a smallish herb with a tough root system. While it is an essential oil in its own right, it is often used as a base oil. It is extracted by steam distillation from the dried fruit.

Carrot Seed has a warm, woody odor that blends well with other spice and wood oils. It is particularly beneficial for skin conditions that relate to nervous tension, such as dermatitis, eczema, psoriasis, or nervous rashes. It also has the added benefit of bringing a restorative quality to prematurely aging skin or mature complexions, restoring vitality.

Traditionally, Carrot Seed was used for its nutrients, as it

GERANIUM for harmony, balance, security, comfort, regularity in menstrual cycle.

is high in vitamins. As an effective tonic, it has a restorative quality on the liver and gall bladder. It is especially beneficial for jaundice complaints or for excessive consumption of alcohol, since it rebalances the kidneys and liver. It is said to stimulate and reactivate kidney function, and is excellent for relieving liver congestion. It can also be used to promote and stabilize the menstrual cycle.

As one of the seed oils, its inherent quality is one of inspiration and vision. Carrot Seed tends to draw out a shy and withdrawn person's personality.

Using this oil, you'll have the opportunity to grow and expand, exploring new activities and experiences.

IT ADDRESSES: Prematurely aging skin, liver disorders, jaundice, scarring, eczema, psoriasis, nervous rashes, irregular menstruation, shyness, despondency, lethargy.

IT HELPS PROMOTE: Courage, inspiration, new ideas and experiences, rejuvenation, balancing of the kidney and liver.

SAFETY INFORMATION: Nontoxic, nonirritating. Do not use during pregnancy.

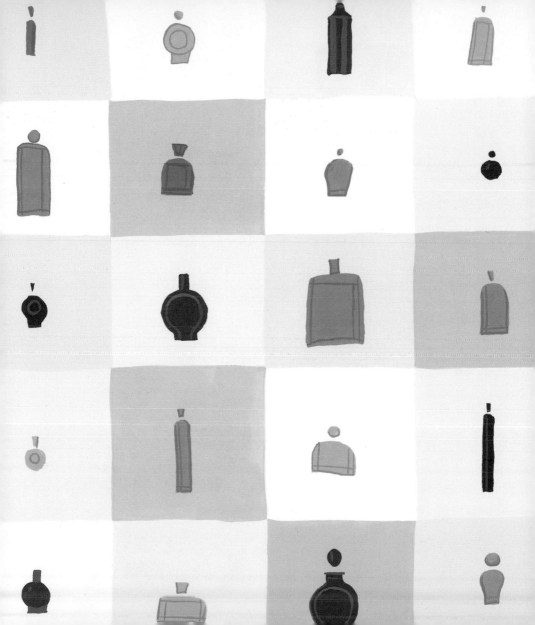

CEDARWOOD (Juniperus virginian)

The cedarwood is a tall, slow-growing evergreen conifer adorned with red-brown cones; it conveys majesty and stature. Judging it from a physical standpoint, you can see how it can bring inspiration, focus, and purpose to your life. The oil, extracted from the leaves, barks, and twigs of the tree, has been used to treat myriad ailments ranging from menstrual disturbances to arthritic and skin conditions.

Cedarwood is known for its effect on the chest and lungs; it fights colds by removing excess fluids in the body. As an expectorant, it can be used for bronchitis and asthmatic problems.

Cedarwood is excellent for skin conditions associated with discharge, such as dandruff and seborrhea. It acts as a restorative oil, alleviating conditions such as eczema and acne. This oil, with its strength and fortitude, is excellent for relieving long-term stress and chronic nervous conditions.

Cedarwood is the oil to use when you want to turn a problem into a challenge. Breathe in its vapors to help you deal with heavy demands on your relationships, either in the workplace or at home. This is the oil to help you conquer difficulties and to reinstate a sense of well-being about your achievements and accomplishments. For endurance and fortitude, it can yield excellent results when used with Black Pepper.

The decon-
gestive nature of this
oil not only affects the lungs,
but also your life experiences, as it
releases congestion and confusion that often
reign when you feel overwhelmed or are faced with
long-term challenges. In situations where you feel alienated,
this oil imparts a sense of wisdom and strength.

The steadying influence of Cedarwood helps you avoid rash emotional reactions when you are feeling threatened or emotionally stretched.
It strengthens and brings restoration and comfort.

IT ADDRESSES: Skin conditions, eczema, acne, dandruff, seborrhea, excess fluids, bronchitis and asthma, arthritis, long-
term stress, chronic nervous conditions.

IT HELPS PROMOTE: Inspiration, focus, purpose, wisdom,
strengthening of the chest area, fighting of infections and colds,
expectorant and decongestant action.

SAFETY INFORMATION: Do not use on inflamed or irritated
skin. Do not use during pregnancy.

CHAMOMILE (German) (Matricaria chamomilla)

This aromatic herb, with featherlike leaves and small flowers, treats the most delicate conditions. German Chamomile is the most anti-inflammatory of all the essential oils, and it is one of the most long-standing medicinal herbs.

This oil is remarkable for addressing irritability, both on a physical and emotional level. Generally speaking, it brings a calming quality to conditions associated with inflammation. On a physical level, it relieves irritated skin and allergic conditions, and immediately soothes general inflammation. To promote healing, apply a Chamomile wash to an open wound or skin fissure. To address the frustration of sleeplessness, especially where children are concerned, a warm Chamomile bath helps.

German Chamomile's deep blue color is due to the high percentage of azulene it contains. This is the most important component that distinguishes it from Roman Chamomile, and it is this characteristic that specifically addresses inflamed conditions of the skin, such as dermatitis, psoriasis, and inflamed joints.

German Chamomile also re-regulates energy centers in the body, as it relaxes the nervous system, relieves any

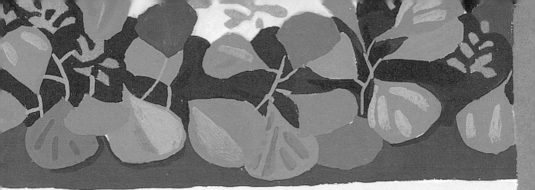

spasm or restriction, and eases pain. It is excellent for insomnia and for any restrictive interferences in the body, such as indigestion, constipation, irritable bowel, and headaches.

It has an antispasmodic, analgesic effect on the body, as it releases muscular spasms; and it is an age-old treatment for menstrual disorders. German Chamomile blends well with Cypress and Clary Sage to treat premenstrual tension and pain.

Its warm and sweet herbaceous odor blends well with other floral oils to bring peace and harmony to the body. Blended with citrus oils, it helps promote a sense of inner peace. As German Chamomile works to relax and calm you, you'll find that you can communicate more fluidly. As anger and frustration are released, more joy flows into your life.

When you're feeling out of control or you think that circumstances have a hold over you, German Chamomile can help settle and calm you, relieving nervous tension.

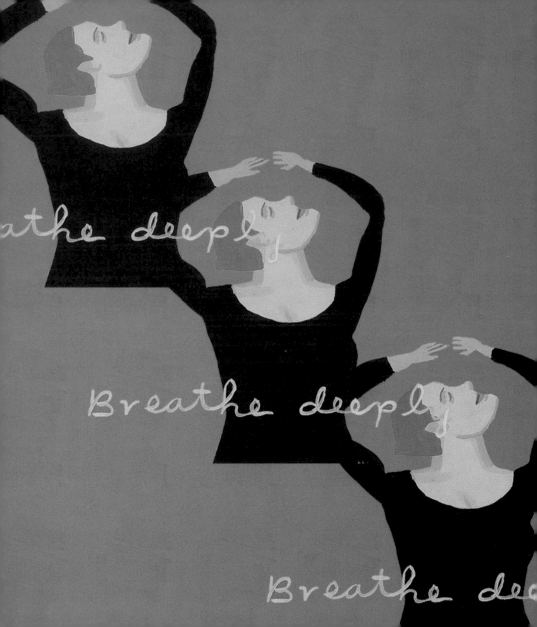

This oil releases the pressure of expectations, setting you free from the restrictions of self-imposed limitations. The more you can support yourself, the more you can help others. German Chamomile promotes calm, ease, and openness.

German Chamomile can help you follow your intuition and be more in touch with what is called your "gut feeling." It is the oil to use to reinstate self-esteem and a sense of self-worth, encouraging you to reach your full potential.

IT ADDRESSES: Irritability, inflammation, allergic and irritated skin, skin fissures, dermatitis, psoriasis, inflamed joints, insomnia, indigestion, constipation, irritable bowel syndrome, headaches, nervous system problems, menstrual disorders, PMS.

IT HELPS PROMOTE: Calm, ease, harmony, relaxation, relief, joy, resolve, muscle ease, self-esteem, self-worth, antispasmodic action.

SAFETY INFORMATION: Nontoxic and nonirritating unless used in a high concentration on inflamed dermatitis conditions.

CHAMOMILE (Roman) (Anthemis nobilis)

This small and stocky herb is often compared to German Chamomile, but grows to only half the size. With many branches and a featherlike leaf system, it tends to spread and creep. Its daisy-white flowers are quite a bit larger than those of the German variety. It is native to Europe and North America and is often cultivated in England and the USA. The essential oil is extracted from the flower head by steam distillation.

In ancient times, Roman Chamomile had a reputation for promoting good health; it was known as "the physician." It is excellent for treating nausea, anorexia, vomiting during pregnancy, and any conditions where there is a disturbance or disruption in the digestive tract. Where digestive disorders are associated with nervous conditions, Roman Chamomile yields great results.

Roman Chamomile possesses an antibacterial quality and has a profound effect on the genital, urinary, and reproductive systems. It is excellent for inducing and regulating menstruation, particularly for women who have painful or difficult periods. Roman Chamomile can be used with Clary Sage for PMS and irritability. As a balancing oil for the female reproductive organs, it can be applied to the abdominal and lower pelvic areas to alleviate conditions such as endometriosis and infertility. It can also be used to rebalance female energies, thus addressing fertility problems.

Roman Chamomile, especially when blended with Lavender, can be used as a wash on acne, boils, burns, cuts, and dry and itchy skin to soothe and calm. It is also beneficial for hypersensitive skin, broken veins, or damaged skin. Add 2 drops to a base cream so it can be used as a moisturizer. It strengthens tissue and is an excellent cleanser for decongesting the skin, especially when there has been irritation.

The aromatic influence of Roman Chamomile is hypnotic, as it relaxes and acts as a mild sedative. This is the oil for rest and relaxation, since it releases anxiety, and reinstates a sense of comfort and belonging. As you release anxiety and fear, patience and peace are revived.

As you free yourself from the restricting emotions of fear and anger, you experience a sense of unconditional love. This oil allows for change and growth, as it unfolds a pathway to peace in front of you.

IT ADDRESSES: Ailments related to the genital, urinary, and reproductive systems; menstruation problems; endometriosis; infertility; acne, boils, burns, cuts, dry, itchy, damaged, hypersensitive skin; broken veins; anxiety; impatience; feelings of restriction; worries.

IT HELPS PROMOTE: Healthy skin, rest, comfort, feelings of belonging, patience, peace, change, growth, sleep, health of the female reproductive organs, clean skin, regeneration.

SAFETY INFORMATION: Nontoxic, nonirritating. Do not use in the early months of pregnancy.

CINNAMON (Cinnamomum zeylanicun)

This exotic evergreen tree grows up to 50 feet tall. Its strong and thick branches are covered with leathery, shiny green leaves with small flowers. The inner bark of the tree is gathered every two years and sold in the form of cinnamon sticks for domestic use; however, this is not the origin of the essential oil, which is extracted from the leaves and twigs of the plant. The warm, spicy aroma and its yellow-brownish liquid are reminiscent of treacle. It is grown in exotic areas and is native to Sri Lanka, Madagascar, the Comoro Islands, Burma, and India, each area tending to produce a specific species.

Cinnamon can be used in a preparation to provide an effective liniment or rub for headaches, rheumatic pains, or muscular stiffness. It brings about mobility and warmth, particularly if the body experiences aches resulting from colds in the cooler months. It is powerfully anti-infectious and addresses infections that can aggravate bronchitis or an irritated throat. An inhalation of Cinnamon can relieve coughs, colds, and sore throats.

The antifungal qualities of this oil can be used in a wash to treat infected skin and wounds, and it acts as a potent astringent to tone and cleanse. Cinnamon is used as a decongestant on the skin, and it is especially helpful for people living in highly polluted environments, or those who have sluggish lymphatic systems.

Cinnamon acts as an aid and tonic to a sluggish circulatory system, and also as a stimulant to the cardiac system to promote vitality and increase energy.

It is excellent for intestinal complaints such as colitis, diarrhea, and dyspepsia, and also for any intestinal parasites that linger on after the infection has gone (or as a result of taking antibiotics). It can be used effectively to address frigidity or impotency, as it revitalizes the body and mind, especially when you're feeling weak or exhausted.

Cinnamon is the oil to use when you're feeling separated or isolated, as you can often become emotionally cold during times like this. Cinnamon alleviates fear, arouses the senses, and stimulates your subconscious mind.

With the use of Cinnamon leaf, energy and vitality are restored, and the bond and connection with others are reestablished. Combine Cinnamon leaf with Black Pepper and Mandarin to revitalize and reawaken the body and mind.

IT ADDRESSES: Bronchitis, coughs, colds, sore throats, infected skin, wounds, the lymphatic system, the circulatory and cardiac systems, colitis, diarrhea, dyspepsia, intestinal parasites, impotency, lethargy, despondency, lack of vitality.

IT HELPS PROMOTE: Mobility, warmth, restoration, vitality, increased energy, antifungal and anti-infectious action, decongestion, cleansing of the skin.

SAFETY INFORMATION: Do not use during pregnancy, or with babies and children under age five. Do not use on sensitive or damaged skin. Apply to the surrounding area of wounds only—not on the wound itself.

CITRONELLA (Cymbopogon nardus)

This plant—a tall perennial grass—has been used for its aromatic and medicinal properties in many cultures throughout the world. Its fragrance suggests that it is of the citrus family, yet it is more closely related to Lemongrass. Often used to treat fevers and intestinal parasites, its active principles serve as a digestive aid.

Citronella has been known to ease pelvic pain associated with menstruation.

It is well known as an insect repellent and room deodorizer, and it has been used for centuries in Eastern countries to cleanse any environment and rid it of unwanted bugs and odors.

Blend with Cedarwood oil for an excellent remedy in the fight against mosquitoes. It works well in the summer months to treat excessive perspi-

Dill +

ration; and in the winter months, it protects the immune system, relieves minor infections, and prevents colds and flus.

Citronella is an antiseptic and antibacterial agent, with the capacity to address rheumatic and arthritic pain. Due to its potent fragrance, it works effectively on the most robust of natures, especially when overwhelming fatigue has taken over the body, or where ongoing stress produces headaches and migraines.

Citronella oil clears and uplifts, bringing about a new sense of self-assuredness. As you awaken to the circumstances that have produced fatigue and exhaustion in the body, you are more able to clear your path. This oil creates a broader outlook for those who have been rigid and unyielding in their perspective on life.

IT ADDRESSES: The immune system, colds, flus, excessive perspiration, fatigue, headaches, migraines, rheumatism, arthritis, loss of confidence, exhaustion, rigidity. It is an insect repellent.

IT HELPS PROMOTE: Openness, self-assurance, a clear head, sensory awareness, clearing out of the old, antiseptic and antibacterial action.

SAFETY INFORMATION: It is nontoxic and nonirritating, but use with caution on extremely sensitive skin or dermatitis conditions. Lemongrass or Eucalyptus may be more suitable for these skin disorders.

CLARY SAGE (Salvia sclarea)

This strong perennial herb grows up to three feet high, has large featherlike leaves colored green with a hint of purple, and small blue flowers. Clary Sage is native to Morocco, the Mediterranean, Southern Europe, and England.

This highly revered herb has for many years been used for digestive disorders and kidney malfunction, and is excellent for the female reproductive organs.

Clary Sage is particularly useful before and during menstruation for alleviating menstrual cramps and uterine contractions. It tends to act as a tonic for the genito-urinary and reproductive systems. This oil is also excellent for amenorrhea (absent periods) and excessive discharge. It can be used with Roman Chamomile to rebalance the female reproductive organs. With its estrogen-like qualities, it stimulates hormones and regulates the cycle. It can be used during labor to ease pain. Clary Sage is the most euphoric of all the essential oils, and as an inhalant, is excellent for postnatal depression. It reduces menopausal symptoms such as hot flashes, mood swings, frigidity, and lack of interest in sex. While it is not considered an aphrodisiac, Clary Sage is certainly an oil that allows for greater intimacy.

Clary Sage is also an excellent oil for whooping cough and asthma, where there is chronic or ongoing wheezing and constriction in the chest cavity. It helps alleviate muscular aches and pains, and spasms and cramps, as it acts on the circulatory system. It has a tendency to lower high blood pressure and can be used for obesity. With high-fat diets, this oil helps lower high cholesterol because it aids arterial circulation.

Clary Sage acts to strengthen and fortify one's mental capacity. It is an excellent oil for the elderly because it eases the fear and paranoia associated with getting older. It is also helpful for those going through a mid-life crisis. In conjunction with Frankincense and Orange, it can help people with extreme fears and nightmares. It can also expand a dream state to enable a more creative and peaceful sleep experience.

Clary Sage acts as an astringent on the skin to address acne, boils, dandruff, and hair loss. It can be used in conjunction with Sage for puffy and oily skin. It is an excellent cell regenerator for mature skin.

Clary Sage relieves fatigue and stress, and helps you become more intoxicated with the joy of life, as opposed to being overwhelmed with the pressures of daily routines. It is excellent for weepiness, absent-mindedness, and emotional instability, having a regenerating and inspiring quality that ensures tranquility. It allows for acceptance of one's worth, and as time unfolds, it enhances one's self-esteem.

IT ADDRESSES: The genito-urinary and reproductive systems, menstrual cramps, uterine contractions, menopause, hot flashes, mood swings, frigidity, asthma, muscular aches and pains, spasms, the circulatory system, high blood pressure, obesity, cholesterol levels, emotional instability, anxiety, nervous tension, feeling overwhelmed.

IT HELPS PROMOTE: Euphoria, intimacy, increased mental capacity, inspiration, self-esteem, health of the reproductive organs, stimulation of the hormones, cell regeneration.

SAFETY INFORMATION: Nontoxic, nonirritating. Do not use during pregnancy. Do not use while drinking alcohol, as it can enhance the narcotic effect.

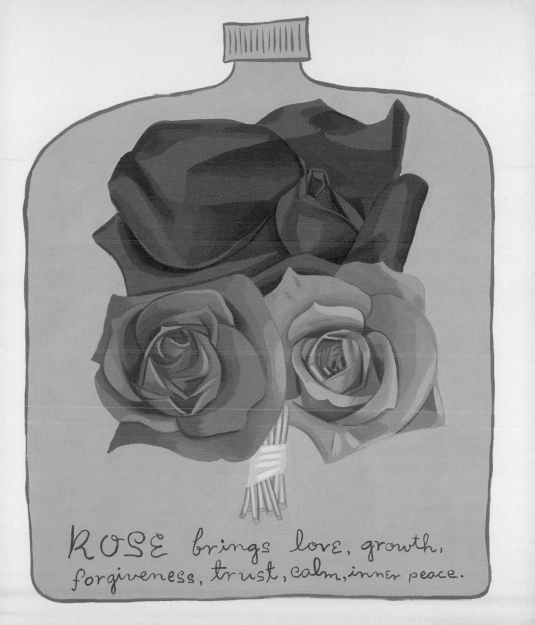

ROSE brings love, growth, forgiveness, trust, calm, inner peace.

CORIANDER (Coriandrum sativum)

Coriander is an annual herb, hardy in stature, that grows approximately three feet high. It has bright green leaves, delicate and dainty white flowers, and small round fruits that turn from green to brown. Native to Europe and Western Asia, it is cultivated throughout the world and used commercially to spice foods.

The coriander seed has been an aromatic stimulant for the past 3,000 years. It is well documented by Greek and Sanskrit writers, as well as the ancient Egyptians, who steeped the seeds to make a potion, and drank it as an aphrodisiac. In the Dark Ages, herbal healers used Coriander to create love magic, and it was often used as an ingredient in a drink served at weddings and festive occasions to raise the spirits, bringing about joy and warmth.

Inherent in this oil is energy and creativity. With its warming qualities, it brings newness to old situations. It is excellent for promoting circulation and for mobilizing muscles and joints, especially in arthritic conditions and for sprains and strains or postoperative healing. Where there is stiffness resulting from injury or poor circulation, use this oil in a massage blend combined with Black Pepper and Lemongrass.

Coriander can be used with Neroli and Lavender to treat stretch marks and scar tissue.

It is an excellent remedy for ailments of the digestive tract. Where there is a nervous condition associated with poor digestion—such as anorexia, muscular spasms, colic, flatulence, or diarrhea—Coriander acts as a mobilizer and helps to balance the system. It is an excellent antispasmodic, and is often used for abdominal distention.

Coriander is a euphoric oil and tends to act as an aphrodisiac, as it warms the body and provides serenity and effective stimulation to calm and uplift the mind. Coriander is excellent in states of nervous depression or instability associated with anxiety or worry.

It is an oil that provides a sense of security, quiets a busy mind, and allows softness and peace to develop. With its stabilizing influence, it helps you enjoy life before rushing on to the next activity.

Coriander can be used in cases of insomnia with Marjoram and Orange, or with Lavender and Jasmine (especially when there is emotional frigidity) to soothe, calm, and surrender.

IT ADDRESSES: Arthritic conditions, sprains, strains, muscle spasms, postoperative healing, insomnia, poor digestion, worry, anxiety.

IT HELPS PROMOTE: Warmth, stimulation, peace, protection, sustenance, security, groundedness, spontaneity, energy, creativity, circulation, antispasmodic qualities.

SAFETY INFORMATION: It is nontoxic and nonirritating, but caution is needed on highly sensitive or damaged skin. Stupefying in large doses.

CYPRESS (Cupressus sempervirens)

This statuesque evergreen conifer can typically grow until it is almost 150 feet tall. While it bears small flowers that eventually produce a round cone, it is usually the fresh, dark green leaves and twigs that contain most of the essential oil. It is native to the Eastern Mediterranean area and is most often distilled in France, Spain, or Morocco.

In Tibet, Cypress is still used today for its purifying qualities, and it is a common incense ingredient. Its characteristic qualities of wisdom and strength are symbols of eternity that continue to inspire the human spirit. The cypress tree, found around graveyards throughout the Mediterranean, is said to be a source of solace for those experiencing grief. The boiling of both its leaves and cones has long been favored for its astringent and binding action. Ancient Assyrians would use this application for curing hemorrhoids.

Years ago, physicians would use Cypress for abnormal discharge—for example, internal bleeding, diarrhea, vomiting, or any excessive "wet" respiratory conditions.

With its antiseptic, anti-infectious qualities, Cypress helps heal respiratory disorders such as sore throats, laryngitis, sinusitis, or bronchitis. It is excellent as an inhalation for whooping cough, sinus infections, flus, colds, and asthmatic conditions. Its antispasmodic quality is effective during asthmatic attacks.

Cypress is a vaso-constrictor used to treat hemorrhoids or varicose veins, as well as skin conditions. Its sweat-producing action, coupled with Sage and Lemon oil and applied as a spritzer to remove excess oils during the day, acts as a powerful skin tonic.

Its ability to harmonize the flow of bodily fluids makes it an important aid for menstrual problems, or for excessive bleeding or discharge from the body. Cypress also aids sluggish intestinal conditions and is a good oil for rehabilitation during convalescence, when the system has been slowed down. It is beneficial in weight-loss programs and assists with excess fluid and water retention in the body, edema, and swelling in arthritic or rheumatic conditions.

Emotionally, Cypress is an oil for excesses and weepiness. It helps rebalance emotions when experiencing sorrow and grief through loss. Often feelings of isolation and frustration can have untold repercussions on the body's physical capacities. Allow Cypress to encourage you to emerge once again and liberate your energies.

Cypress is beneficial for taking control of your life and moving forward, as opposed to expending your energy in the past. It cleanses and purifies the spirit, and is used with Lemon for children when they need protection and stability.

IT ADDRESSES: Sore throats, laryngitis, sinusitis, bronchitis, whooping cough, colds, asthma, hemorrhoids, varicose veins, menstrual problems, excessive bleeding, excess fluid, water retention, edema, arthritic swelling, grief, loss, sorrow.

IT HELPS PROMOTE: Cleansing, purification, protection, stability, taking control, moving forward, anti-infectious and antispasmodic action.

SAFETY INFORMATION: Nontoxic; not irritating or sensitizing. Do not use during pregnancy. Do not use with conditions associated with high blood pressure.

DILL (Anethum graveolens)

This is an annual herb that grows to approximately three feet high.

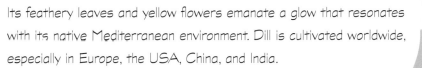

Its feathery leaves and yellow flowers emanate a glow that resonates with its native Mediterranean environment. Dill is cultivated worldwide, especially in Europe, the USA, China, and India.

Dill has always been used as a digestive aid. Its antispasmodic qualities greatly assist the digestive process. If you've indulged in rich and heavy foods, you'll find Dill helpful in stimulating digestion. A blend can be used on the abdominal cavity to relieve colic conditions in young children. This oil can be used for children from early on, particularly with digestive and respiratory ailments, and especially when the whole plant has been extracted—as opposed to the seeds only.

For those with a delicate stomach associated with nervous conditions, Dill allays emotions in order for digestion to take place. When blended with Rosemary and Juniper, Dill acts as an excellent cleanser for the entire intestinal region. A sluggish colon tends to manifest in depressed and sad moods; Dill can be used to mobilize stagnant and repressed emotions, while exercising a mobilizing action in the colon.

As an effective diuretic, it can be used in cases of obesity and water retention. It soothes and supports the kidneys, particularly when blended with Sandalwood for its anti-inflammatory action.

Dill, used with Eucalyptus and Lemon as a chest decongestant, is helpful for those suffering from lung complaints. In

conjunction with Myrrh and Tea Tree, it is excellent for alleviating viral infections.

Dill can be used in combination with Neroli for those who feel emotionally unbalanced, especially when there have been emotional shocks. It helps activate awareness, especially in those who are interested in expanding their consciousness. The paradox is that Dill has the faculty of gentleness, yet is a pungent and potent source of nature.

The eternal cycles of regeneration are inherent in the qualities of this oil, as they assist in processing and reinventing. Those who have fear or disillusionment about the natural processes of life can benefit greatly from the use of Dill, as it revitalizes vision and dissipates challenges.

Dill removes expectations, while at the same time promoting a profound awareness of possibilities.

IT ADDRESSES: Disillusionment, disappointment, oversensitivity, stagnant and repressed emotions, water retention, obesity, the digestive tract, colic, lung complaints, viral infections.

IT HELPS PROMOTE: Mobility, awareness, regeneration, revitalization, vision, vitality, rebalancing of emotions, diuretic and anti-inflammatory actions.

SAFETY INFORMATION: Do not use for frigidity or impotency, as it may depress sexual energy. Do not use on sensitive skin. Should not be applied when going out in direct sunlight.

EUCALYPTUS (Eucalyptus globulus)

This tall and gracious evergreen grows up to 300 feet high. It is native to Australia and is also cultivated in Spain, China, and Portugal. The mature tree produces young blue-green leaves from which the essential oil is extracted. There are hundreds of species of Eucalyptus, of which at least 500 produce essential oil.

Eucalyptus has been extensively researched and has long been used for treating respiratory conditions. Historically, in Australia, the

Say an affirmation

dried leaves were smoked as tobacco to alleviate asthmatic and bronchial conditions when the oil or medicinal preparations were not available. Eucalyptus water has been used in oral applications to treat viruses and bacterial conditions in the body.

Eucalyptus acts as a powerful expectorant and decongestant, due to its balsamic effect; and helps to condition the lungs, strengthen the respiratory tract, and alleviate colds. When treating respiratory disorders, it blends well with Tea Tree, Cedarwood, and Myrrh.

While on vacation or spending time in open environments, use Eucalyptus as an insect repellent in conjunction with Basil and Citronella. It can also serve as a remedy for head lice in conjunction with Tea Tree and Thyme, simultaneously treating skin infections.

When soaking in a bath, muscular aches and pains benefit from the use of Eucalyptus. It is an excellent aid for poor circulation, especially during the winter months. In conjunction with Lavender and Juniper, it works well in a topical application for arthritic and rheumatoid conditions, and is commonly referred to as an antiviral oil. Eucalyptus activates the oxygen exchange in the skin cells and promotes radiant skin.

Its primary action, opening the lungs and healing the body,

also benefits a congested mind, so use this oil as an inhalant to clear the head and help with focus and concentration.

This oil encourages the body to better utilize oxygen, so you can take in life more fully and revive the spirit. Revitalizing you at the deepest level, it promotes a sense of confidence and encourages you to see a broader picture, eliminating restrictions or negative feelings. This oil can give you "room to breathe."

IT ADDRESSES: The respiratory tract, asthma, bronchitis, colds, bacteria, viruses, skin infections, arthritis, rheumatism, lethargy, lack of oxygen, exhaustion, insect problems.

IT HELPS PROMOTE: Oxygenation, revitalization, new opportunities and perspectives, revival, radiant skin, a clear head, focus, concentration, antiviral action, decongestion, clearing of the lungs.

SAFETY INFORMATION: Nontoxic, nonirritating. Do not use during pregnancy.

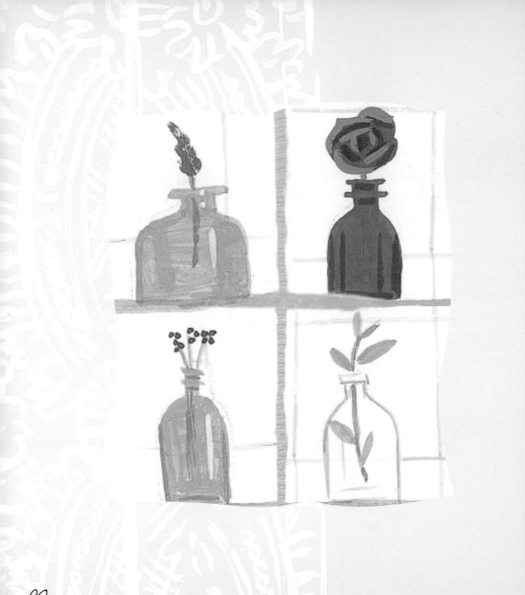

EVERLASTING (Helichrysum italicum)

As an aromatic shrub, Everlasting grows to a height of just under two feet and has delicate yellow flower heads. These flowers rarely wither; therefore, this plant is often referred to as Immortelle. Native to the Mediterranean region, it grows profusely in Italy, France, and Spain, and is also found in Yugoslavia.

On a therapeutic and medicinal level, this essential oil has a profound effect as an antispasmodic on the respiratory and cardiovascular systems. It is anti-inflammatory and anti-microbial, and tends to act as a powerful antiseptic on the body. When dealing with an "itis"—any sort of inflamed condition—it soothes and calms, and it has the ability to reduce inflammation. Everlasting is best used with German Chamomile and Lavender when there is heat in the body.

This is an oil that promotes a sense of immortality. It is excellent for use when there is trauma to the skin, body, and emotions. To address injury or bruising, it is best used with Juniper. Everlasting heals dermatitis and allergic conditions of the skin.

To mobilize the major systems of the body, especially the lymphatic and circulatory systems, Everlasting is best used in warm baths and in massage blends. It tends to alleviate any congestion in the body leading to headaches, migraines, or muscular aches and pains.

Preferably treat these conditions in a bath or by inhalation.

With its potent antispasmodic and cold-fighting effects, Everlasting can be used in conjunction with Cypress and Cedarwood for respiratory conditions such as asthma, bronchitis, sinusitis, chronic cough, and whooping cough. On an emotional level, it can be used to treat chronic stress conditions such as migraines, depression, and debilitation.

This oil, with its energizing and pleasing sensations, deeply affects blood circulation, bringing vitality and fluidity to the whole circulatory system. It also eases the pain and restriction of rheumatic and arthritic conditions. Due to its ability to promote circulation, it is useful in cases of broken capillaries or venous conditions.

Where the body has been wounded or the emotions assaulted, this essential oil provides relief. With its profound psychological effect on the rise and fall of emotions, it has the capacity to mobilize emotional paralysis; as a result, some irritability and frustration may occur. Everlasting is an oil that comforts, alleviates stress, softens the blow of shock and hysteria, and mobilizes suppressed emotions.

Everlasting is an oil of compassion, inspiring tenderness and kindness. Compassion brings understanding, allowing others to support and encourage you. With its capacity to decongest, unblock, and regenerate, this oil acts as a brilliant tonic for the body, mind, and spirit.

IT ADDRESSES: Discouragement, mental congestion, aggression, lack of compassion, irritability, bruising, hemorrhaging, scarring, sprains, strains, neuralgia, inflammation, respiratory discomfort and ailments, congestion due to colds, toxins in the body.

IT HELPS PROMOTE: Understanding, support, calm, peace and ease while sleeping, dream activity, healing to damaged skin, regeneration, strengthening of the immune system, lymphatic drainage and cleansing.

SAFETY INFORMATION: Nontoxic; not irritating or sensitizing.

FENNEL (Foeniculum vulgare)

Fennel is a perennial herb that often grows to approximately six feet tall. From its leaves, a golden yellow flower is produced. The two types of Fennel, bitter and sweet, grow in different regions. One is native to the

ROSE brings love, safns trust, calm, in forgiveness, trust, calm, in

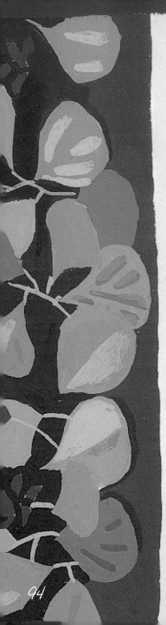

Mediterranean, and is found growing wild in France, Spain, and North Africa. This is often cultivated in Hungary, Bulgaria, Germany, France, and Italy. The sweet Fennel, on the other hand, has primarily been grown in France and Italy.

Fennel has many ancient medicinal applications. It was said to sustain one's vitality and youthfulness, and at the same time, bring about a sense of moral courage and fortitude. This was because it was considered to support self-expression and productivity, and unlock one's potential.

On a physical level, the principal qualities of Fennel affect the digestive tract where, once applied, it acts as an antispasmodic on the intestinal muscles and relieves indigestion, bloating, and flatulence. In the lower abdominal cavity, it also assists with conditions of stagnation such as constipation. It has a regulating action on the digestive and respiratory systems, has the ability to clear sinuses when you have a cold, and can assist in allaying the effects of asthma.

Fennel can induce menstruation and ease menstrual cramps. It assists in labor because it supports the natural process of childbirth. In conjunction with Lemongrass, it has the capacity to increase milk flow. However, caution is necessary—since they are both potent, aromatic oils, it is advisable to use this blend around the breast area only, but avoid use while actually breast-feeding.

Due to its mild diuretic properties, Fennel supports the lymphatic system as a decongestant and tonic, while acting as a cleanser, ridding the body of unwanted fats and fluids. Fennel, coupled with Rosemary and Juniper, helps control obesity and water retention, and also combats cellulite.

Fennel oil encourages you to be more productive, and more conscious and aware of your changing relationships. With its warm and sweet aroma, Fennel helps unleash creative expression.

This is an oil that inspires moral courage and self-expression. With its purifying, cleansing, and invigorating actions, it prevents stagnation, unleashing a more productive way of thinking in an overactive mind.

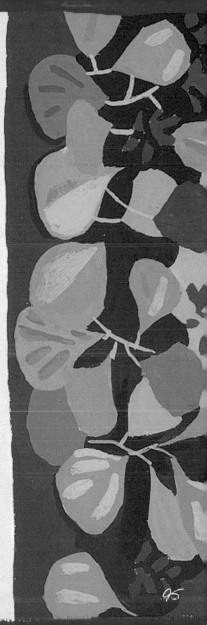

With its keen ability to reestablish and support natural body rhythms and flow, Fennel can be used to promote sexuality or full sexual expression.

IT ADDRESSES: The digestive tract, bloating, flatulence, constipation, congestion due to colds, asthma, menstruation, cramps, childbirth issues, obesity, water retention, cellulite, insecurity, lack of enthusiasm, pessimism.

IT HELPS PROMOTE: Purifying, cleansing, or invigorating actions; new possibilities; self-expression and creative qualities; ease of labor; increased milk flow; healthy female reproductive organs; circulation.

SAFETY INFORMATION: Not irritating. Do not use on highly sensitive skin, on epileptics, or during pregnancy. Avoid contact during breast-feeding.

FRANKINCENSE (Boswellia carteri)

A small tree that grows to a height of 10 to 20 feet, Frankincense displays white-pink flowers with narrow and abundant foliage. The

Smooth

essential oil is taken from the resin, which is collected by making an incision in the bark of the tree; the gum is thus collected to distill the essential oil. It is native to Middle Eastern countries, Northern Africa, and warmer climates. It is also found in Somalia, Ethiopia, Arabia, China, and Lebanon, although the distillation of the resin often takes place in Western countries such as the U.K., Europe, and the USA.

Frankincense played an extensive role in the religious life of the ancient Egyptians and Romans. It was one of the gifts borne to baby Jesus by the three wise men, and it is said to connect you to your higher self.

Frankincense is renowned as an aromatic incense, and its ritual, cosmetic, sacred, and aromatic functions were enjoyed by the Egyptians, who used it in the embalming process.

Medicinally, it serves to treat and heal wounds, inflammations, and skin disorders. Frankincense has the capacity to regulate and strengthen the respiratory tract and helps to open the chest and heart region, especially when used with oils such as Cedarwood, Myrrh, Jasmine, and Lavender. It has a "drying-up" effect on the sinuses when blended with Cypress.

Its wide and extensive use in the cosmetic and fragrance

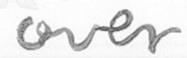

industry is founded on its capacity to act as a skin tonic, as it helps to heal wounds and scars, and to promote a regenerative quality for mature skin.

In traditional applications, you can discover its link to your modern-day life—Frankincense provides a fundamental connection to ritual and sacredness. Its capacity to calm and quiet the mind brings a sense of deep tranquility and establishes a profound connection to the higher self. Frankincense helps you unfold your potential and brings about awareness of your true purpose.

Frankincense heals old wounds on both a physical and emotional level, and assists in overcoming grief and emotions that repress your creativity. Frankincense alleviates fear when the irrational feelings overcome your sense of confidence. It can be used for preventing and eradicating nightmares. When you are emotionally exhausted, Frankincense gives you insight into what is needed to help you move forward. It deepens your belief in the divine, strengthens your convictions, and links you to the eternal.

IT ADDRESSES: Grief, panic, anxiety, paranoia, fear, dehydrated skin, cuts, abscesses, acne, boils, poor circulation, muscular aches and pains, asthma, bronchitis, nervous tension.

IT HELPS PROMOTE: Tranquility, openness, transcendence of the ego, connection to the higher self, acceptance, awakening to new possibilities, rejuvenation of the body and mind, healing of the skin, strengthening of the lungs.

SAFETY INFORMATION: Nontoxic but sensitizing. Do not use during pregnancy.

GERANIUM (Pelargonium graveolens)

This bushy shrub with its heart-shaped leaves and dense pink flowers grows to about three feet high. There are over 200 different species, most of which are found in Southern Africa and widely cultivated in Russia, Egypt, Japan, Central America, and Europe. While the plant is native to these countries, the essential oil production itself is usually conducted in four major regions—

Egypt, Russia, China, and an island near Madagascar called Reunion.

Traditionally, Geranium has been used in all forms of herbal medicine, and as a remedy, it dates back many hundreds of years. Its principal properties were used to overcome ailments such as dysentery, as well as those conditions associated with the reproductive system, such as inflammation and excessive bleeding. Therefore, Geranium is still used today as a remedy and resource during menstruation to balance the cycle. It can be used to alleviate menopausal symptoms; and to balance highs and lows, irritability, and mood swings. Challenges associated with birth can be helped through the use of this essential oil.

As an everyday application, Geranium is excellent for treating skin conditions associated with bruising, dermatitis, ulcers, eczema, psoriasis, or whenever regeneration, rejuvenation, or healing is needed. As a wash or in a cream, it is an excellent skin-care aid.

In conjunction with Frankincense and Cypress, Geranium can be used to alleviate asthma, balancing the chest, and clearing mucus. It is also beneficial in an aromatic bath for rheumatism and osteoarthritis. It acts as a tonic for conditions of poor or restricted circulation, such as hemorrhoids. It stimulates the lymphatic system and provides an excellent aid for the immune system.

Geranium helps establish a sense of personal security and intimacy. It can be used to support postnatal blues, bringing harmony and

receptivity to challenges that arise with the welcoming of a new baby.

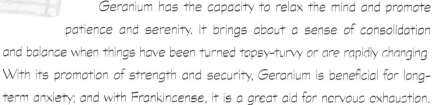

With its anti-inflammatory qualities, Geranium works on a physical and emotional level to reduce and quiet inflamed emotions and skin.

Geranium has the capacity to relax the mind and promote patience and serenity. It brings about a sense of consolidation and balance when things have been turned topsy-turvy or are rapidly changing. With its promotion of strength and security, Geranium is beneficial for long-term anxiety; and with Frankincense, it is a great aid for nervous exhaustion.

IT ADDRESSES: Acne, eczema, dermatitis, excessively oily skin, inflammations, rheumatism, mosquito bites, wounds, prebirth labor, postnatal blues, menstrual cramps.

IT HELPS PROMOTE: Balance, security, certainty, regeneration, comfort, harmony, cell renewal, regular menstrual cycles, balance during menopause, recovery after plastic surgery, balancing of emotions, healing of the body.

SAFETY INFORMATION: Nontoxic; not irritating or sensitizing. Do not use during pregnancy.

GINGER (Zingiber officinale)

This medicinal spice is native to Asia and is one of the oldest spices used in cooking and culinary delights. The essential oil is extracted from the root. The oil is mostly distilled in the U.K., China, and India. It is a native of Asian and tropical environments.

In herbal folklore, Ginger was used medicinally for its warming qualities and to treat conditions such as rheumatism, muscular aches and pains, fatigue, and joint injury. It was especially beneficial for ailments of the lower back.

Inherent in a root oil is its capacity to draw up nutrients from the ground; thus, Ginger is an excellent digestive aid and can be used over the abdominal cavity to mobilize the digestive process, cleansing the body and purifying it of toxins. It is beneficial to use when you have overindulged in either food or alcohol. It is also excellent for diarrhea and colic, and can be used with Roman Chamomile for loss of appetite and anorexia.

During the winter months, the warming qualities of this oil can assist and promote circulation to the extremities of the body, warming toes and fingers. It makes an excellent remedy for colds, chronic bronchitis, congestion, and coughs, as it counteracts infections. Blend with Eucalyptus to combat sinusitis and sore throats.

It strengthens the kidneys and helps relieve lower back pain, especially when associated with nervous conditions or long-term injury.

Ginger has a fiery nature and helps you develop and strengthen confidence and willpower. In ancient China, it was used to treat male impotency and is still known today as an aphrodisiac. It activates sexual energy and promotes a sense of confidence and esteem when initiating a new relationship or becoming more intimate.

Ginger fortifies, stimulates, clears the head, diminishes the tendency to procrastinate, and encourages you to move away from self-doubt. Use it with Basil and Lime for decision-making and focus, as it can make you more vigorous and sustains energy levels.

Ginger sharpens the senses, opens the mind, and gives you a potent sense of exhilaration.

IT ADDRESSES: Bruises, congestion, bronchitis, fatigue, muscle injury, loss of memory, constipation, diarrhea, migraines, headaches, infections, impotency, frigidity, self-doubt, lethargy, coldness.

IT HELPS PROMOTE: Confidence, courage, awakening of the senses, full sexual expression, exhilaration, good circulation, regular menstruation, proper digestion and colon function.

SAFETY INFORMATION: Nontoxic. Do not use on sensitive or broken skin. Do not use in direct sunlight.

GRAPEFRUIT
(Citrus paradisi)

This citrus oil originates from a tall, strong tree that explodes with large yellow fruits and is found extensively in tropical Asia, the West Indies, California, Florida, Brazil, and Israel. The essential oil is taken from the peel of the fruit. It is commonly used in the perfume and cosmetic industries because of its refreshing and energizing aroma. Most Grapefruit is produced in California.

Like other citrus fruits, Grapefruit has an ability to tone your system and prevent infection because of its antiseptic quality. It has a beneficial effect on the respiratory system, helping to decongest. This oil can also cleanse the liver and digestive tract, and is excellent for use in weight-loss programs since it is a diuretic—that is, it alleviates water retention—and it breaks down fat in the body. It is a lymphatic stimulant and helps regulate the circulatory and lymph systems, simultaneously detoxifying the body. Take this oil to the gym so you can use it after you've exercised, because it eases muscle fatigue and stiffness and tends to help clear lactic acid from the body.

Grapefruit, like other members of the citrus family, helps tone oily or acne-prone skin. It decongests clogged pores and tightens the skin, promoting a livelier complexion. It stimulates hair growth when combined with Rosemary and Cedarwood, and is excellent for use during the colder months when moods are depressed and the body feels constricted. It restores vitality and lightens the spirit.

If you tend to use food to feed your emotions, Grapefruit is an excellent oil to have in a vaporizer or daily massage blend to discourage this type of eating. It clears congestion, eases frustration, and is primarily a clarifying oil that eases prolonged anxiety and alleviates disappointment connected with unfulfilled expectations. Use this oil to uplift, impart confidence, and revive the spirit.

IT ADDRESSES: Oily skin, blocked pores, acne, hair loss, muscle fatigue, stiffness, obesity, cellulite, bulimia, a toxic liver, infections, fluid retention, feeling overburdened, frustration, disappointment.

IT HELPS PROMOTE: A cheerful and positive outlook, joy, spontaneity, cooperation, clarity, a cleansed liver, muscle ease and responsiveness, detoxification.

SAFETY INFORMATION: Nontoxic, nonirritating. Phototoxic—do not use in the presence of UV rays.

HYSSOP (Hyssopus officinalis)

A warm and sweet aroma emanates from this perennial, evergreen shrub, which grows up to two feet in height. A purple-blue flower is displayed from the woody stems and slender green leaves of the Hyssop bush. The oil is most commonly obtained from Germany, France, and Italy, while the plant itself is native to the Mediterranean region and temperate areas of Asia. It grows wild throughout the USA, Russia, and Europe; and is also culti-vated in Hungary, France, and Yugoslavia.

Hyssop has a particularly volatile nature, which suggests, both in herbal traditions and in modern-day applications, that it's most beneficial to the respiratory system because it regulates and decongests. It has an astringent effect on the skin, and as a tonic it can be used to regulate the nervous system, especially when stress leads to skin conditions.

The Romans used Hyssop for its purifying qualities, to protect themselves against the Plague, and to disinfect when medicines and other aids were not available. From ancient times, famous healers used this herb for its expectorant action on the chest and lungs. In

Enjoy the

Enjoy the calm

Enjoy the cal

Hebrew practices, Hyssop was used to purify ceremonial and religious environments; thus, the Hebrews refer to it as a holy herb symbolizing spiritual cleansing.

Hyssop strengthens the lungs and restores vitality to a deficient immune system; however, it must be used with caution because it is a hot oil and extremely stimulating. It eliminates physical debilitation, as it opens the chest, energizes the circulatory system, and energizes the entire mind/body connection.

Not too dissimilar to Thyme, Hyssop can be used for its expectorant action in conjunction with Eucalyptus and Tea Tree to treat bronchitis, sinusitis, and congestion; or in the winter months for colds, flus, and viral infections.

Hyssop is a restorative oil that alleviates conditions of depression, melancholy, lethargy, and very specifically, pessimism.

It has the capacity to protect, and benefits those who are feeling particularly vulnerable to the environment and to the pressures of day-to-day life.

It addresses: Liver disorders, intestinal parasites, viruses, flus, colds, debility, sinusitis, bronchitis, asthma, inflammations, fungal infections, congestion, liver function, depression, anxiety, lack of vitality, despondency, poor concentration, fatigue.

It helps promote: Alertness, wakefulness, awareness, expansion, purification, strength of body and mind, good circulation, respiration, digestion.

Safety information: Not irritating or sensitizing. Do not use during pregnancy.

JASMINE (Jasminum officinale)

This evergreen vine, with its delicate star-shaped flowers, exudes an exotic aroma. Native to China, North India, and West Asia, it has been cultivated along the Mediterranean coast, California, China, and India. There are many

species of Jasmine, and traditionally this plant has been used for medicinal and perfumery applications. In China, the flower was used for conditions of the liver, such as cirrhosis and hepatitis, as well as dysentery.

This is the oil to use to dispel fears and warm the heart. Jasmine has been widely used in the East, and in India is often referred to as the "Queen of the Night" because its scent is much more potent when the sun sets. In Indian mythology, the Hindu god of love, Kama, is said to have tipped his arrows with Jasmine blossoms in order to pierce the heart with desire. Jasmine was used in ancient times to perfume the air on special occasions and has often been seen as a symbol of love and longing.

It acts as a mild analgesic and has a *carminative* effect on the gut—that is, it expels gas. As an expectorant, it affects the lungs as it cleanses and supports the respiratory system. It relaxes the body so it can be used to treat muscular spasms and sprains.

Its main application is on the genito-urinary system, where it was traditionally used in herbal medicine for painful periods and to regulate and stabilize uterine disorders. It is particularly useful in treating the reproductive system, especially when there has been an impact on fertility and potency through nervous dispositions or trauma.

Jasmine calms the nervous system and releases tension, and it is one of the most potent essential oils for addressing restlessness and chronic depression. Its warming and restorative action imbues an environment with joy, unleashing creativity and giving birth to new ideas.

It is known for its use as a fertility herb and is a potent aphrodisiac, as it brings warmth and sensuality to your physical being while encouraging you.

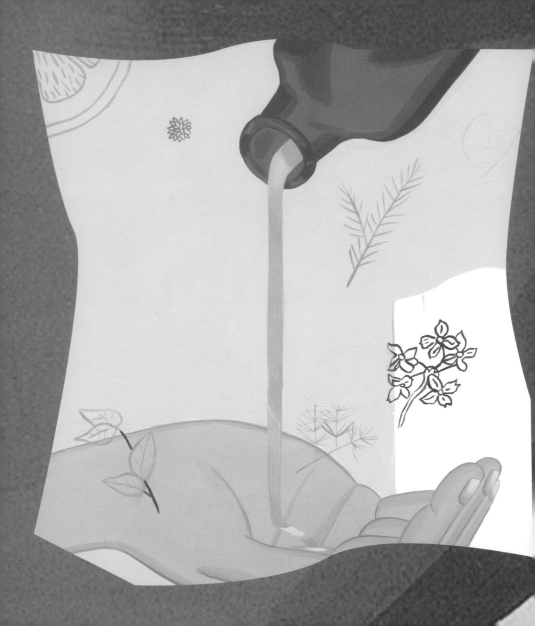

Jasmine reassures, warms, and awakens passions.

Coupled with Frankincense and Marjoram, it is an excellent oil to combat nightmares, paranoia, and fear. By itself, Jasmine builds confidence and alleviates emotional suffering.

> IT ADDRESSES: Sensitive skin, muscular spasms, sprains and strains, congestion, coughs and colds, laryngitis, sleeplessness, the genito-urinary and reproductive systems, nightmares, fears, impotency, lack of sexual desire, restlessness, emotional frigidity, trauma.

> IT HELPS PROMOTE: Desire, passion, sensuality, confidence, assertiveness, optimism, self-esteem, ease in childbirth, a regular menstrual cycle, deep relaxation, ease in respiration.

> SAFETY INFORMATION: Nontoxic; nonsensitizing.

JUNIPER (Juniperus communis)

The juniper tree is an evergreen with blue-green, pinelike needles. The essential oil is extracted from its berries. While native to Northern Europe, Southeast Asia, and North America, the main production takes place in Italy, France, Yugoslavia, Spain, Germany, and Canada. There are up to 60 species of Juniper. Traditionally, the needles and berries were used for medicinal application, predominantly to treat urinary infections, and these qualities are still known to be effective today. In a body-rub blend, Juniper can be used to address urinary infections such as cystitis and urethritis. Along with activating the kidney and bladder functions, it acts as a potent diuretic and reduces water retention in the body. Due to its effect on the kidneys, bladder, and urinary system, Juniper alleviates chronic tiredness that may be associated with fluid retention.

You can also use Juniper for cellulite, since it breaks down toxic matter in the body. It also aids lymphatic circulation. Due to its cleansing action, Juniper is effective for arthritic conditions, especially when there has been injury or stiffness in the joints. Juniper mobilizes the joint, aiding in the repair of the tissue. In cold and damp environments, Juniper brings about warmth and mobility. Where there is warmth and activity, healing occurs, and the mobilization of the restricted joint is soon apparent.

Juniper is an anti-infectious remedy for cold conditions when there is wheezing and congestion, such as bronchitis, asthma, and whooping cough. In conjunction with Geranium and Cedarwood, Juniper is excellent for treating skin conditions such as dermatitis or eczema, and also treats oily skin. It's effective as a facial wash, refreshing and energizing the skin.

Juniper helps you move through emotional exhaustion and listlessness, bringing activity and strength to your everyday life. It is an oil of empowerment, helping you cleanse and purge the past. It stimulates openness and a sense of inner vision and support.

For those feeling weak, or during convalescence, this oil strengthens and uplifts. In combination with Frankincense and Sandalwood, Juniper inspires centeredness and is valuable during meditation.

IT ADDRESSES: A toxic lymphatic system, obesity, rheumatism, arthritis, fluid retention, oily skin, hair loss, dermatitis, painful or absent periods, colds and flus, immobility, congested emotions, emotional exhaustion, disempowerment.

IT HELPS PROMOTE: A sense of self-worth, strength, and conviction; purification and purging; toning of the skin; mobility to the joints; cleansing of the body; the opening of the mind.

SAFETY INFORMATION: Nontoxic and nonsensitizing. Do not use during pregnancy. Should not be used with conditions associated with kidney disease.

GERANIUM for harmony, balance, security, comfort, regularity in menstrual cycle.

LAVENDER (Lavandula angustifolia)

This evergreen shrub, with its fragrant flowers, grows to a height of about three feet. Its slender stalks with narrow feathery leaves and purple flowers are taken to produce the fine aroma of true lavender. It is predominantly found throughout the mountainous areas of the Mediterranean countries. The main producers of this popular essential oil are France, Bulgaria, Yugoslavia, Italy, and England. There are many species of Lavender, but therapeutically, True Lavender is the most important, whereas Spike Lavender is often used in perfumes and cosmetic preparations.

In ancient folklore and traditional herbal texts, Lavender is well documented as a reputable healer. It has always been used to comfort, and it is known to revive the spirit and calm the mind.

For general health, Lavender can be used as tonic water. In air-conditioned environments, where heat and constricted levels of oxygen tend to activate nervous anxiety, this oil can be used to address faint-headedness, palpitations, and giddiness, as it soothes and calms the nervous system. It certainly is an "essential" essential oil!

Lavender is excellent during convalescence in postoperative and palliative hospital care. It relieves fatigue and makes a wonderful first-aid remedy for trauma and hysteria, as it has restorative properties.

On the skin, it has a profound action as a cell stimulant; and it can be used for acne, eczema, psoriasis, and bruises. It is a valuable aid when healing scar tissue, thread veins, wounds, burns, or ulcers on the skin. It is also beneficial for allergic conditions, activating cell renewal at the deepest level.

Lavender can be used in any blend when taking care of a nervous disposition or a physical disorder such as muscular spasms, nervous asthma, and bronchitis triggered by severe nervous anxiety. It is a cardiac tonic and helps lower high blood pressure; therefore, it can be used when caring for the elderly.

Acknowledged for its fresh, soft, and calming influence, Lavender has earned a reputation as the "mothering oil." In times of crisis or when comfort is needed, this oil brings about composure and stability. It calms strong emotions when you're feeling threatened or fearful.

It is excellent for treating insomnia, and a few drops on the pillow at night calms the most restless baby.

When you're committed to breaking old patterns, this is the oil to use. It eases the trauma of change. Lavender diffuses frustration and irritability so that the opportunity for full expression is presented.

Lavender is the oil of serenity and composure. It opens you to new ideas and allows you to let your inspiration guide you to new heights.

IT ADDRESSES: Asthma, respiratory complaints, a nervous disposition, bronchitis, muscle spasms, strains, bruises, psoriasis, burns, scars, damaged skin, wounds, scarring, painful periods, headaches, convalescence, insomnia, exhaustion, impatience, frustration, irritability.

IT HELPS PROMOTE: Serenity, composure, self-expression, gentleness, rest, spirituality, compassion, radiant skin, digestion, ease in childbirth, sound sleep, rejuvenation of body and mind, comfort, security, a sense of general well-being, cell stimulation, healing, repair of the skin.

SAFETY INFORMATION: Nontoxic; not irritating or sensitizing.

LEMON (Citrus limonum)

This small evergreen tree grows to almost 20 feet high. Just one tree can produce as many as 1,300 lemons per year, making it one of the most abundant fruit-producing trees.

Similar to other citrus trees, this one originated in Asia. It grows in East India and the Mediterranean regions; and is also found in Spain, Portugal, and Italy. As a sun lover, it is now produced in North America.

All parts of this fruit have been used for their medicinal values—the peel to perfume gloves and to repel insects, the juice and inner fruit for their antiviral properties. In ancient times, it was also used to prevent the onslaught of scurvy for sailors who spent many months at sea. Particularly in European countries, Lemon became a cure for infections of the body and was said to be beneficial for clearing up bacteria.

Due to its clarifying and detoxifying action, Lemon is a powerful remedy that can help decongest the chest. Its antiviral action helps it work on colds, coughs, and flus in the winter months, especially when these ailments have been triggered by overwork and a weakened immune system.

Lemon supports the body as a tonic, and it is effective in ridding the body of phlegm and congestion. It assists in weight reduction and stimulates the lymphatic system, making it an excellent oil for treating cellulite and obesity. It can also be used to treat high blood pressure associated with these conditions.

Coupled with Grapefruit, Lemon helps decongest a toxic liver. At the same time, it alleviates conditions that are often associated with an overworked liver, such as nausea, headaches, irritability, and insomnia.

As a therapeutic agent, you can rely on Lemon's astringent properties and its energetic nature to improve circulation and tone capillaries and veins. It also assists with conditions such as hemorrhoids and nosebleeds, when combined with Cypress in a base oil.

Lemon is one of the most beneficial oils for clearing the head, regaining focus, and restoring trust. Since it refreshes and uplifts, it can transform a congested and overburdened mind, dissipating confusion. It helps ease worry and fear, encouraging intuitive thought. Lemon provides a sense of assuredness. It is an oil to use during decision-making, especially when fears have held you back in the past. This oil allows you to trust yourself more fully and uplifts and reconnects you to those things that are most important.

IT ADDRESSES: Congestion due to colds, infections, respiratory disorders, infected skin, slackened muscle tissue, poor circulation, low blood pressure, nosebleeds, a sluggish lymphatic system, coughs, obesity, stomach acidity, confusion, a lack of purpose and direction.

IT HELPS PROMOTE: Certainty; clarity; direction; sharpened awareness; sensory acuity; vigor; vitality; trust; purpose; focus; muscle and skin tone; venous strength; good circulation, digestion, and liver function.

SAFETY INFORMATION: Nontoxic. Do not use in the presence of direct sunlight or UV light. Do not use during pregnancy.

LEMONGRASS (Cymbopogon citratus)

This perennial tropical grass grows rapidly to reach a height of nearly five feet. Its distinctive lemon fragrance smells similar to that of the citrus family, although it is an herb and not a citrus plant. Lemongrass is a sought-after ingredient in perfume and cosmetic preparations. It is native to Asia, specifically West and East India, and is also grown in Madagascar. It has traditionally been used in Indian medicine for infections and fevers, and even today, Lemongrass has been proven to act as a sedative on the nervous system.

Its potent qualities assist the workings of the digestive tract and stimulate gastric juices, as it is beneficial for the stomach. It helps regulate the autonomous nervous system and acts as an analgesic for headaches and migraines, especially when caused by a nervous disposition or digestive disorder.

It makes an excellent massage treatment, since it eases muscular spasms, sprains, and strains. Take Lemongrass to the gym for a post-training rubdown, as it improves muscle tone and disperses lactic acid throughout the body. Its capacity to relieve muscular aches and pains is of great benefit after a heavy day at the office when tension needs to be relieved—place a few drops in a warm bath. The potency of the aroma works

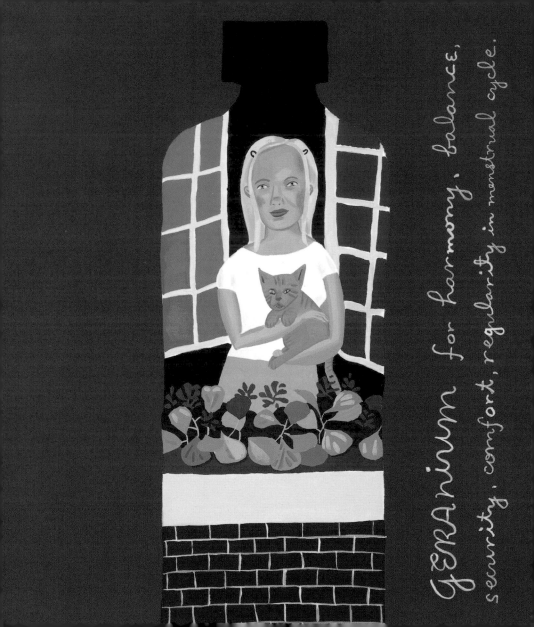

GERANIUM for harmony, balance, security, comfort, regularity in menstrual cycle.

as an effective mobilizer for robust people who have become lethargic and despondent. It is extremely beneficial for stress-related conditions and for use during times of nervous exhaustion, as it energizes the senses yet soothes the body.

Lemongrass is an excellent deodorizer in the home, due to its effective antimicrobial action. It is a particularly powerful oil for use on strong or offensive body odors. Lemongrass acts as a refreshing sanitizer.

In conjunction with Lavender, Lemongrass makes an excellent tonic for the immune and lymphatic systems, promoting blood flow. It energizes you in the morning if you're feeling lethargic and fatigued.

The mobilizing influence of Lemongrass, while regenerating and rehabilitating, also allows for inner growth and development. When you feel regenerated, anything is possible. As pathways open, use Lemongrass to sustain the momentum in creating something new.

IT ADDRESSES: Depression, lethargy, despondency, moodiness, inflammation, parasites, bacteria, cellulite, dehydration, a toxic lymphatic system, arthritis, muscular sprains, strains, aches and pains, loss of vital energy, despondency, depression, fatigue.

IT HELPS PROMOTE: Concentration, energy, vitality, mobilization, activity, strength, sustenance, a healthy immune system, muscle tone, support to the connective tissue, good liver function, deodorization.

SAFETY INFORMATION: Nontoxic. Dermal irritant, especially on sensitive skin. Do not use on open skin. Do not use during pregnancy.

LIME (Citrus aurantifolia)

Lime is a small evergreen shrub that grows to approximately 15 feet high. Lime has a sharp spine, smooth leaves, and white flowers. Its fragrance is sharp and bittersweet. Lime originated in Asia and is cultivated in many warm countries, notably Italy, where citrus fruits are popularly grown. It is also cultivated in Florida, the West Indies, and Central America. It grows naturally in tropical environments. There are several species of Lime, and it is the bitter Lime that is used for medicinal applications.

Lime oil shares many attributes with Lemon oil. Traditionally, it has been used for similar purposes: for fever and infections, and as a chest rub for coughs and colds during the colder months. It is also an excellent aid for indigestion and dyspepsia, as it assists in allaying the discomfort of over-acidity in the stomach. It can be used in a massage blend for rheumatic conditions, as it has an antiviral effect on the body. It can also be used as a restorative tonic and pick-me-up.

Lime is an excellent source of vitamin C. It acts as a disinfectant and astringent on the skin, is beneficial as a deodorizer for sweaty bodies, and can be used as an astringent for oily, greasy skin.

As a chest rub, it breaks down congestion; alleviates symptoms of colds and flus; and eases coughs, sore throats, and strains to the respiratory tract. It combats infection and is a great preventive oil.

As with many of the citrus oils, Lime is a wonderful digestive aid, and for those who suffer from loss of appetite, it encourages hunger by activating digestive juices.

Due to its sharp and stimulating effect, Lime is an excellent oil for those who are feeling bored or apathetic toward life. For those suffering from depression, listlessness, and exhaustion, it refreshes, uplifts, stimulates, and brings a cheerful demeanor to the most despondent mood.

Lime helps establish a sense of enthusiasm about life, creating energy and eagerness when starting new projects. It brings a sense of delight and excitement to your life, producing a rippling

ROSE brings love, trust, calm, inspo, forgiveness,

125

effect on those around you. Lime is an oil for encouragement, clarity, and lightheartedness.

It is also a restorative oil and can be used to treat alcoholism due to its energizing and clarifying effects on the mind and body.

IT ADDRESSES: Rheumatism, coughs, colds, congestion, infections, muscle spasms, sore throats, viral infections, digestive disorders, loss of appetite for food and life, low concentration, lack of direction, listlessness.

IT HELPS PROMOTE: Cheerfulness, optimism, enthusiasm, energy, clarity, vitality, liver function, muscle tone, toned skin, cleansing, stimulation.

SAFETY INFORMATION: Dermal irritant and sensitizer. Should not be used on sensitive skin. Do not use during pregnancy. Do not use in the presence of UV light or on damaged skin.

MANDARIN (Citrus recticulata)

Native to Southern China, this small evergreen tree can grow more than 20 feet high. With deep green, glossy leaves and fragrant flowers, the tree bears the sweet mandarin orange fruit in abundance. Mandarin oil, being citrus, is expressed from the peel of the fruit, and due to its delicate and most inviting aroma, is regarded as one of the most important oils in massage. It is mainly produced in Italy, Spain, Algeria, Cypress, Greece, the Middle East, and Brazil; and more recently, in the tropical climes of Florida and California.

Especially in Europe, Mandarin is a traditional favorite for children due to its gentle effect on the digestive system and liver function. The essence of Mandarin is a symbol of the inner child.

Mandarin acts as an antiseptic in the body and also has an anti-spasmodic effect on muscles. Being a cardiovascular tonic, it promotes circulation. It also assists with intestinal problems and digestive disorders. In contrast to many of the other citrus oils, Mandarin is sweet, with a floral undertone. It helps to sedate, and quiets and calms those suffering from insomnia.

Mandarin stimulates the appetite and activates the liver, acting as a tonic for the digestive tract. It helps break down fats in the body and aids in the secretion of bile. Since it calms the intestinal environment, it assists in expelling gas from the body.

Due to its uplifting qualities and its capacity for relieving tension, it is an excellent oil to use in combination with Clary Sage and Geranium for PMS and menstrual cramps.

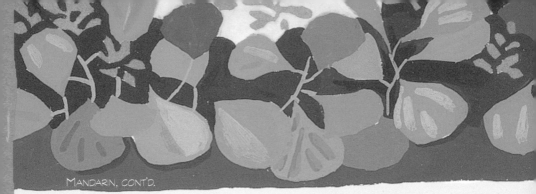

This oil brings a sense of comfort to those who find themselves rigid or stuck. It assists in redefining your truth, and establishes a unity between body, mind, and spirit. When you experience Mandarin's joyous and radiant qualities, you'll find it easier to move forward in relationships and environments that have been somewhat defined or inflexible. This oil brings more love and light to everything you do.

IT ADDRESSES: Stretch marks, scars, dry skin, dehydration, muscle spasms, bronchitis, cardiovascular disorders, flatulence, indigestion, a toxic liver, menstrual cramps, PMS, depression, insomnia, rigidity, grief, rejection, trauma.

IT HELPS PROMOTE: Inspiration, tranquility, lightness of being, radiance, the emergence of the inner child, sound sleep, muscle ease, a healthy liver, a good appetite.

SAFETY INFORMATION: Nontoxic; not irritating or sensitizing. Should not be used in the presence of UV light.

MARJORAM (Origanum marjorana)

Sweet Marjoram originates in Egypt and throughout Mediterranean regions, and nowadays is mostly obtained from France and Spain. It is also grown in Egypt and North Africa; and is produced in Tunisia, Morocco, Bulgaria, and Germany. The essential oil is distilled from all parts of the plant, which tends to grow to a height of almost two feet. It is a bushy perennial with dark green oval leaves and small white flowers. Its botanical name, Origanum, is derived from the Greek word meaning "joy of the mountains."

Marjoram has traditionally been used as a perfume, cosmetic, and medicinal ingredient. The Greeks use wild Marjoram as a funeral herb; it is planted around graves to ensure that peace and harmony dwell with the parting spirit.

Marjoram is extremely versatile in its aromatherapy applications. It has a soothing, stabilizing, and warming effect on the emotions and the body, and is a valuable aid for menstrual disorders. This oil possesses a rare quality—it strengthens and calms simultaneously. Its tendency is to tone and clear as it calms the mind. It is a powerful antispasmodic and analgesic for the chest, and is particularly beneficial for muscular stiffness, aches, and pains.

It can be used for intestinal colic, flatulence, and to soothe the gut. In conjunction with Ylang Ylang, it is an excellent oil for palpitations, tachycardia, and states of hypertension, as its antispasmodic actions serve to alleviate these conditions. It also clears the chest of congestion, while strengthening the lungs.

During the winter months, it brings about warmth and inspires activity. Blend this oil with the oxygenating oil Eucalyptus for chronic lethargy during the winter months.

It is the most effective of all the essential oils for insomnia. Marjoram serves to relax, unwind, and free the mind so that sleep is unhindered. Marjoram is an oil for respite and repose; it restores and balances you.

Marjoram is known to be an anti-aphrodisiac, and can be used when there is high sexual energy in a professional or personal environment, quelling the sexual appetite.

It assists in regulating the menstrual cycle, alleviating painful menstrual cramps. In conjunction with Basil and Lime, Marjoram is especially beneficial for PMS.

Marjoram is one of the most versatile and helpful essential oils. It tends to eliminate feelings of persecution and victimhood. It is most useful in times of grief, since it restores an inner sense of assuredness, calm, courage, and confidence. It is particularly beneficial for those suffering from a deep trauma or heartache. When experiencing the loss of a loved one, Marjoram helps you accept your loss and allows an inner sense of worthiness and self-esteem to come to the fore. It nourishes an inner knowing; and allows restoration to take place in the heart, mind, and body.

IT ADDRESSES: Coughs, respiratory disorders, restricted breathing, muscle spasms, nervous bronchitis, respiratory distress, infections, bronchitis, muscular stiffness, arthritis, rheumatism, chilblain, bruises, palpitations, colds, flus, hypertension, constipation, irregular or painful periods, excessive sexuality, low self-worth, disconnection, grief.

IT HELPS PROMOTE: A sense of certainty, security, peace, calm, sincerity, perseverance, confidence, celibacy, clear skin, a fortified nervous system, the autonomic nervous function, stress relief.

SAFETY INFORMATION: Do not use during pregnancy. Do not use on asthmatic conditions. Due to its sedative qualities, do not use when low blood pressure exists. Do not use for depression or with depressed people.

MELISSA (melissa officinals)

This Mediterranean plant, most commonly grown in France, exudes a sweet lemonlike aroma. It grows to approximately two feet high and is soft and bushy with a bright green, serrated leaf. The flowers of the plant grow in small loose clusters and are usually white, pink, or yellowish. Native to the Mediterranean, it is cultivated in gardens the world over and has been acknowledged from time immemorial for the delight that it inspires, aromatically and medicinally.

The analgesic and antispasmodic properties of Melissa have been well reported and documented by Arabian physicians such as Avicenna in the early 11th century, who recorded that the balm made the heart merry and joyful, strengthening the spirit. Its reputation for benefiting heart and nervous conditions was long ago associated with the widely held opinion that Melissa could promote longevity. Paracelsus, a

Swiss-born physician, referred to Melissa as "the elixir of life." This is an oil that does not come cheap; therefore, beware of inexpensive imitations. Only a very small amount of oil is derived from the distillation of this plant.

Melissa has also been used to regulate the menstrual cycle and promote fertility. Applied as part of a massage blend over the abdominal and pelvic girdle, it helps balance and regulate reproductive functions.

Whenever the cardiac system or the circulatory system has been overstimulated, Melissa acts as a tonic and balm to ease stress, and release the spasm and fatigue that can be associated with these conditions. Its close affinity with the female reproductive system helps to create regularity and balance. It also acts as a tonic for the uterus.

With its calming effect on emotions and especially on hypersensitive states, Melissa is an excellent aid for releasing the intensity of migraines and headaches. In conjunction with Lavender and Neroli, it is said to be of great benefit for states of hysteria.

Melissa can be used in conjunction with Basil to treat migraines, or with Lavender and Marjoram for insomnia. It eases nervous anxiety and tension, preparing the body for slumber.

Melissa dispels fears and helps sustain energy levels during times of rapid change, shock, or grief. It dissipates anger, bringing a deeper sense of understanding and acceptance to the underlying issues in a relationship or experience.

In conjunction with Lemongrass, it is effective as an insect repellent. Melissa's hardy nature, yet subtle and soft fragrance, brings these qualities to body and mind. It promotes strength and calmness, allowing you to better express inner feelings of hurt or anger. Melissa restores clarity and brings security, and for those who feel dependent, it brings about a sense of reassurance.

Melissa helps you establish an innocent, childlike quality, while dismissing vulnerability, fear, and distrust.

IT ADDRESSES: Migraines, menstrual pain, nausea, insomnia, restlessness, agitation, trauma, allergic skin conditions, wounds, infections, muscle spasms, rheumatism, asthma, bronchitis, high blood pressure, palpitations, excitation, nausea, menstrual pain, infertility, depression, stress, infidelity, sadness, lethargy.

IT HELPS PROMOTE: Acceptance, understanding, peace, balance, spiritual vitality and growth, clear skin, strengthening of the lungs, toning of the muscular system, circulation, a regular heartbeat, stabilizing of the circulatory system, protection against infection, good digestion, balance in reproductive organs.

SAFETY INFORMATION: Nontoxic; not irritating or sensitizing.

MYRRH (Commiphora myrrha)

Myrrh oil is extracted from the gum that exudes from a species of myrrh tree grown in the Middle East, Northern India, and North Africa. It often reaches a height of 30 feet, with sturdy knotted branches, deeply aromatic leaves, and small white flowers. The trunk exudes a pale yellow resin that hardens to a semitransparent gum, called the "tears of the tree" by those indigenous to the countries in which the tree grows.

In antiquity, this gum was one of the first substances treated as precious, and valued for its enduring scent. Myrrh played an intrinsic role in the religious and medicinal life of the ancient Egyptians. It was the main ingredient of perfumes, cosmetics, and agents used for embalming and healing. It was used to treat conditions such as arthritis, menstrual problems, sores and wounds, and leprosy.

Myrrh is known for strengthening the chest area—specifically in asthmatic conditions—as well as for treating coughs and colds; ridding the body of congestion; and as a preventive measure against sore throats, mouth ulcers, and wounds. Myrrh oil is reddish-brown and viscous, suggesting a warmth and richness for the body. In ancient texts, Myrrh was brought to the Christ child by the Magi, and was used as an essence to connect people to their divine purpose. Today, Myrrh is still used for its ritualistic and sacred properties.

Myrrh oil works powerfully on the emotions; it generates confidence and awareness for those who feel unable to speak up and speak out.

With its astringent qualities, Myrrh can also be used for chronic diarrhea and vaginal discharge. Research has demonstrated that Myrrh helps reduce cholesterol and is therefore the most effective oil for dealing with hypertension and obesity caused by a fatty and toxic diet. Myrrh is well known for its anti-bacterial properties and anti-inflammatory action, and has been used as an expectorant on the chest and throat area.

Used in a vaporizer during meditation, Myrrh helps purify your environment, prepares you for the unfolding of inner wisdom, and helps you accept new teachings and awareness. It is said to enhance visualization and provide you with a sense of freedom as you are released from the mundane and ordinary.

Myrrh helps close old wounds, both physical and emotional, especially those that continue to expel toxic waste from the body. Myrrh oil cleanses, purifies, and soothes. It helps you slow down, meditate, and be peaceful. It allows you to retreat from the hustle and bustle of everyday life and deeply connect to your inner wisdom, securing you in your own power of solitude and resourcefulness.

IT ADDRESSES: Inflamed skin, boils, ulcers, athlete's foot, weeping or prematurely aged skin, sore throats, asthma, bronchitis, coughs, colds, mouth ulcers, diarrhea, degenerative processes, the absence of menstruation, vaginal discharges, emotional weakness, loss of spiritual connection, isolation, emotional wounds.

IT HELPS PROMOTE: Spiritual and inner strength, healing, visualization, a sense of deep connection, psychic capacities, expanded vision, inner peace, resourcefulness, health and preservation of the skin, regeneration, stimulation of white blood cells, balance to the reproductive system, sexual appetite.

SAFETY INFORMATION: Nontoxic, nonirritating. Do not use during pregnancy.

NEROLI (Citrus aurantium)

While this essential oil is extracted from a bitter orange tree, it is not bitter. With its beautiful floral bouquet, it is taken from the fragrant white flowers of an evergreen tree that grows to approximately 30 feet high. It is native to the Far East. The countries that produce orange blossom oil are Tunisia, Italy, Morocco, Egypt, the USA, and France. Tradition has it that this oil was named after the Princess of Nerola in Italy, who adored it as a perfume.

In cultures where orange blossoms have been worn as bridal head-dresses, Neroli was said to symbolize the virtues of purity and virginity. Together with Lavender, Bergamot, and other citrus oils, it has been used as a classic ingredient of eau de cologne.

Neroli's medicinal properties were valued as a tonic for the nervous system, as it soothed and calmed those who became agitated or frustrated. Neroli eases restlessness, insomnia, emotional stress, and tension. Its fragrance is quite hypnotic, and, therefore, tranquilizing to the sympathetic nervous system.

Because of its capacity to regenerate the skin, Neroli assists in treating thread veins, broken capillaries, and stretch marks. It also revitalizes the skin after it has been exposed to excessive sunlight, or when it is affected by stress and tension.

Neroli helps strengthen the respiratory tract, specifically to increase muscle tone and support the respiratory and musculo-skeletal systems. It is a cardiac tonic and promotes circulation, especially to arteries, as it balances and regulates blood pressure.

With its sweet aroma, Neroli blends well with Orange and Lavender to soothe an agitated or hyperactive child. Its calming effects help send children into a deep and relaxed sleep.

Neroli has the capacity to allay irrational fears connected to sexuality, and can encourage receptivity to loved ones.

Neroli helps balance menopausal symptoms, irritability, and frustration connected with PMS. In conjunction with Lavender and Cypress, this is the oil to use when feeling weepy and highly emotional. It helps allay the intensity, and restabilizes.

Neroli expands your sensory acuity, reconnecting you to your own sense of self-worth.

IT ADDRESSES: Broken capillaries, scars, stretch marks, sensitive skin, bronchitis, slackened muscles, circulatory disorders, postoperative care, diarrhea, intestinal discomfort, colic, lack of sexual interest, impotency, depression, PMS, sadness, disappointment, insomnia, shock, lack of self-worth.

IT HELPS PROMOTE: Peace, release, spiritual connection, joy, reassurance, hope, physical and emotional regeneration, elasticity of the skin, strength of the heart, deep sleep.

SAFETY INFORMATION: Nontoxic; not irritating or sensitizing.

NIAOULI (melaleuca viridiflora)

Niaouli is a member of the Melaleuca family, a large tree that grows abundantly in Australia and nearby New Caledonia. Its aromatic scent, pointed linear leaves, and yellow flowers are a familiar sight in New Caledonia. The essential oil is mainly produced in Australia, where it is a native plant and has typically been used in folk and herbal medicine for a variety of ailments, ranging from respiratory disorders to infections.

The antibacterial and antifungal qualities of Niaouli make it an excellent aid in treating viral conditions—specifically in the respiratory tract—and circulatory disorders. As an inhalant, Niaouli can be used to treat infectious lung conditions, and is especially beneficial in easing the pain and congestion of sinusitis. It helps to rid the body of congestion by acting as a powerful expectorant, and has often been used as a mouthwash and throat gargle for infections. In combination with Orange and Eucalyptus, it is an effective freshener in smoky environments.

Niaouli stimulates muscle tone and is therefore great at the gym to use as a preparatory balm for physical activity. In preparation with Tea Tree and Eucalyptus, Niaouli is wonderful as a liniment on muscle spasms or muscular restrictions in the body, specifically when associated with rheumatism and arthritic pain.

Niaouli is a stimulant and a tonic for the digestive tract, and works powerfully on the circulatory system. For a sluggish liver, use in conjunction with Grapefruit oil, as it promotes activity and also cleanses the digestive tract of intestinal parasites.

Use Niaouli for compresses on oily and greasy skins in conjunction with Cypress and Lemon. It cleanses and decongests greasy skin, acne-prone areas, and skin infections. It has a potent regenerative property that increases cell regeneration, and simultaneously helps oxygenate the tissue.

Niaouli is also said to act as a potent aphrodisiac, specifically stimulating male hormonal action and addressing impotency.

IT ADDRESSES: Muscular aches and pains, circulation, rheumatism, acne, boils, burns, insect bites, oily skin, asthma, bronchitis, colds and congestion, urinary tract infections, lethargy. Specifically useful for males.

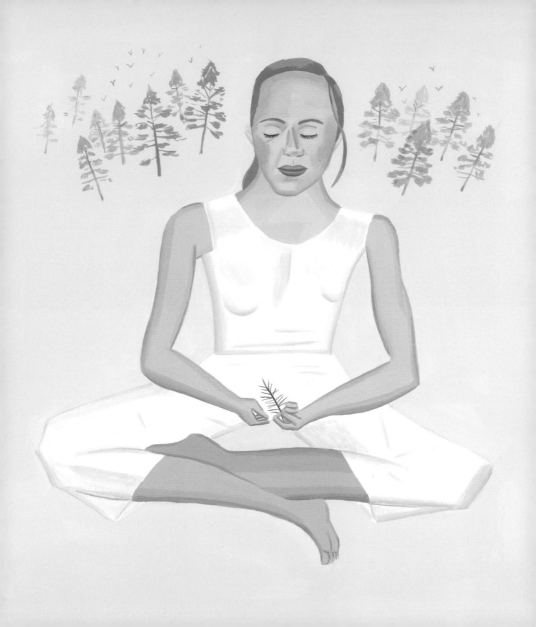

IT HELPS PROMOTE: Mental alertness, male hormonal action, fortification of the immune system, alleviation of colds, strengthening of the mucous membranes.

SAFETY INFORMATION: Nontoxic; not irritating or sensitizing. Do not use during pregnancy or with babies and children under age eight.

NUTMEG (myristica fragrans)

The sharp and spicy aroma of Nutmeg permeates the tropical environments in which it grows. This evergreen tree can grow to more than 60 feet tall, producing a dense foliage with a small yellow flower. A fleshy fruit is contained within the nutmeg's shell and seed, which is distilled to extract the essential oil. Native to the Moluccas, it is cultivated in Indonesia, Sri Lanka, and the West Indies. The oil is distilled widely in the USA, and is utilized for culinary purposes.

Nutmeg has been used for centuries to invigorate and prevent digestive disorders and kidney problems. In Asian countries, It was used to strengthen and tone uterine muscles when applied to the belly. Nutmeg strengthens the cardiovascular system, as it grounds and calms you.

Being a spice oil, its inherent quality is to activate and mobilize; thus, it brings warmth and activity to joint stiffness caused by arthritis or rheumatism. Where there is poor circulation, Nutmeg applied in a topical application mobilizes and stimulates.

In conjunction with Peppermint or Fennel, it is a great aid for flatulence, indigestion, and nausea. It activates a sluggish digestive system when heavy and fatty meals have been eaten.

Nutmeg helps protect the immune system when you're in a toxic environment or unfamiliar circumstances and need to protect against bacterial infections. Its stimulating effect activates and promotes sexual desire, addressing frigidity and impotency. Nutmeg alleviates nervous fatigue, especially when associated with sexual inhibition. It invigorates and activates the body when added to a warm bath, releasing muscular aches and pains, especially where rheumatism or arthritic conditions are apparent. It is also an excellent tonic for the hair.

Nutmeg stimulates nerve impulses and brain activity. When you feel a sense of failure and a loss of vitality, use Nutmeg to reinforce your strength and to encourage and support your endeavors.

It addresses: Arthritis, gout, muscular aches and pains, poor circulation, rheumatism, colitis, neuralgia and bacterial infections, overeating, frigidity, impotency, a sense of loss or failure.

IT HELPS PROMOTE: Sexual enthusiasm and expression, intimacy, liveliness, vitality, sharpened senses, a healthy appetite, the workings of the reproductive system, muscular comfort.

SAFETY INFORMATION: Nontoxic; not irritating or sensitizing. Do not use during pregnancy.

ORANGE (Citrus aurantium)

Having originated in Eastern Asia, the orange tree is one of many evergreen citrus trees, and it is most famous for its juice. The sweet orange tree varies slightly from its relation, the bitter orange, in that it is smaller, less hardy, and the shape of its leaf is stalklike rather than heart shaped. It is now found extensively throughout the Mediterranean region, France, Spain, Italy, Florida, and California. The oil is produced mainly in Brazil, North America, and Italy. It is renowned for its vitamin content and has been used traditionally in Chinese medicine to treat coughs, colds, and anorexia. The orange peel was used to make soaps and cosmetics in England around the 16th century, and today is still a favorite for its sweet and zesty fragrance.

Dr. Moray, who gave rise to the application of massage in

aromatherapy, considered Orange oil excellent for toning the stomach, as an antispasmodic, and helpful for digestion. It also reinforces the immune system and is a natural blood purifier, acting as a good tonic for the body.

If you look at the peel itself, it reminds us of certain skin conditions, so you can remember its usefulness for combating cellulite when you massage it into the skin daily with Cypress and Rosemary. It is also of great value as an after-sun wrinkle treatment.

After heavy meals, Orange is an excellent way to detoxify the system. It also serves as a good mouthwash for remedying bad breath.

Due to its potential to uplift and refresh, Orange helps combat fatigue, premenstrual tension, and stress conditions. During menopause, it can be used for depression. It also assists the body in relieving edema and water retention. Orange has a healing effect on sore muscles, muscle strains, and sprains.

It is good for eczema and dermatitis, helping to rejuvenate the skin; and with Neroli and Sandalwood, it works well on the nervous system as a tonic. Orange also clears out toxins and decongests the skin, encouraging it to look more clean, fresh, and hydrated. Orange is said to help with the formation of collagen and is vital for the repair of body tissue. It softens and strengthens the outer layers of the skin, and stimulates the nerve endings, which activate circulation. It is excellent for stretch marks and helps repair broken bones. Orange acts as a digestive aid for the liver, and it increases and encourages the flow of bile, improving the assimilation of fats.

Orange is quite helpful in the treatment of insomnia. It is deeply relaxing, and coupled with Lavender, can alleviate frustration. It is an oil for spontaneity, encouraging you to handle things with ease. It helps you get out of your head and into your heart, to have more fun, express your love, and engage more fully in life.

IT ADDRESSES: Dry, dull, congested skin; dehydration; cellulite; stretch marks; obesity; edema; constipation; a toxic liver; sore muscles; nervous tension; insomnia; boredom; rigidity; lack of creativity; hopelessness; obsessive behavior; sadness.

IT HELPS PROMOTE: Cheer, clarity, joy, physical well-being, hydrated skin, regeneration, mobility in body functions, revival of spontaneity, communication, warmth in relationships.

SAFETY INFORMATION: Nontoxic, nonirritating. Do not use in direct sunlight or in the presence of UV light.

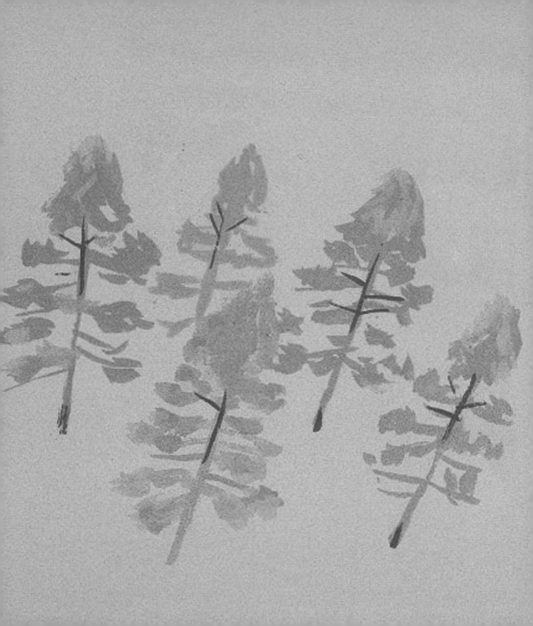

OREGANO (Origanum vulgare)

This plant is often referred to as wild Marjoram, and while it is a member of the same family, its characteristics are quite different. Both of these herbs have traditionally been used for culinary purposes and are often confused. Oregano grows until it is approximately 1 1/2 feet tall. It has purple-pink flowers and bears oval-shaped leaves.

Back in the 13th century, Oregano was used in monasteries for its potent effect on chest disorders and complaints. It was utilized extensively in cooking because of its antispasmodic qualities, which promote the digestive process. It acts as a carminative on the gut—that is, it expels gas—and it can also be used as an operative, so it is an excellent oil massaged into the skin before going out to enjoy a sumptuous meal.

Oregano calms intestinal spasms, especially when the condition is impacted by nervous anxiety. It stimulates the liver and can be used effectively with Orange and Grapefruit. It is also a stimulant for the appetite.

Today, Oregano is still reputed to have a beneficial action on the entire respiratory system, as it works effectively on asthma, colds, bronchitis, congestion, and whooping cough.

It alleviates rheumatic and muscular pain and has an antibacterial and antiseptic effect on the body. Oregano is a potent tonic when used as a preventive oil when going into harsh conditions, or where there is uncertainty about sanitary conditions.

Oregano revives your senses, is a nerve tonic, and is beneficial for migraines because it dissipates the intensity of the pain and pressure. It offers a feeling of well-being and conveys a sense of movement, while simultaneously encouraging you to be more active, energizing your body.

IT ADDRESSES: Rheumatism, asthma, bronchitis, congestion, liver complaints, digestive disorders, rigidity, uncertainty, doubt, listless-ness, lethargy.

IT HELPS PROMOTE: Revival of the senses, clarity, openness, mobility, a sense of vigor, the workings of the respiratory system, antibacterial action.

SAFETY INFORMATION: Can irritate the skin and mucous mem-brane. Do not use during pregnancy. Must be highly diluted for use in aromatherapy. Do not use on babies, young children, or those with sensitive skin.

PALMAROSA (Cymbopogon martinii)

This wild herbaceous grass with its long and slender stems is cultivated before its flowers appear, and the oil is obtained from the fully dried grass.

Indigenous to India, this oil has been distilled for hundreds of years for its culinary and medicinal applications. It is also produced in the Comoro Islands and Madagascar. Palmarosa has always been used commercially to perfume soaps and cosmetics because it is far less expensive than Rose oil, as it has a hint of Rose in its aroma.

Throughout India, Palmarosa has been taken internally and applied externally as a preventive measure against infections and fever. It is an excellent antibacterial and also stimulates the digestive system and alleviates the discomfort of colds, flus, and fevers. It is a digestive aid and can be used to treat anorexia.

In the cosmetic industry, Palmarosa is used as a remedy for healing the skin, which is attributed to its natural antiseptic components. It can work to heal old acne scars and is predominantly used by those who love the sun. For skin that is prematurely aging, it helps smooth out wrinkles and heal broken veins. Simultaneously, it restores balance to the skin, as it regulates oil secretions and is particularly useful for cell regeneration. It is well reputed for its ability to cleanse the skin of general infections such as acne, eczema, and dermatitis.

Palmarosa is an oil for undernourished or dehydrated skin, especially during travel. Its cooling and anti-inflammatory qualities make it an excellent treatment to soothe nervous conditions or alleviate long-term stress associated with flagging skin.

With its anti-infectious properties, it treats bronchitis, sinusitis, coughs, and colds; and it also stimulates the circulatory system. In conjunction with

Eucalyptus, it is excellent for viral infections.

Palmarosa tones the uterus and can also be used in conjunction with Tea Tree to treat thrush, cystitis, and vaginitis.
Along with Marjoram and Orange, it is an excellent remedy for
restlessness and insomnia, as it eases tension and physical exhaustion,
allowing for a restful slumber.

The aromatic grass is mobile and adaptable, and its watery nature conveys a sense of fluidity. This is the quality that it brings to your mind and
emotions. Adaptability often goes hand-in-hand with being nonjudgmental and
releasing expectations. Coupled with Orange for spontaneity, Palmarosa oil
helps foster a sense of acceptance and a tendency to let go.

IT ADDRESSES: Colds, flus, fevers, digestive disorders, anorexia,
acne scars, broken veins, dehydrated and mature skins, bronchitis,
sinusitis, coughs, viral infections, thrush, cystitis, vaginitis, insomnia.

IT HELPS PROMOTE: Restful sleep, mobility, adaptability, fluidity,
grace, anti-bacterial and anti-inflammatory actions, antiseptic
action, good digestion, cell regeneration, cooling.

SAFETY INFORMATION: Nontoxic; not irritating or sensitizing.

PATCHOULI (Pogostemon cablin)

Patchouli grows to a height of approximately three feet. With its sturdy stem, it is a bushy perennial herb that exhibits fragrant flowers, white with a tinge of mauve. It is native to Southeast Asia and grows wild in areas such as Sumatra and Java. It is also widely distributed in the regions of India, China, and South America. The oil is distilled from the dried leaves of the plant, which is harvested either two or three times each year. The leaves are picked by hand and have long been used in the East to scent home environments and prevent disease.

Medicinally, Patchouli is used to treat colds, headaches, nausea, vomiting, and areas in the body that are constricted in some way by muscular pain or spasms. It is an excellent anti-Inflammatory and anti-infectious oil, and is particularly beneficial in treating skin conditions such as dermatitis, acne, cracked or dried skin, wounds, and any injured skin. As a cell regenerator, it is best blended with Palmarosa and Lavender to assist in healing. It can be used on weeping skin in conjunction with Juniper and Geranium to cleanse and heal the skin. It is also excellent during menopausal sweats. With its antibacterial and antiviral properties, it can be used to treat acne, herpes, and chest congestion.

With its warm and earthy fragrance, Patchouli is particularly beneficial for those who suffer from deep depression. It is excellent as an aid during convalescence, as it energizes and warms the senses, energizing and arousing the body. It is of benefit to those with poor circulation and a weakened immune system, especially if there has been chronic anxiety and overwork.

Patchouli arouses passion and can be used as an aphrodisiac because it energizes your enthusiasm for intimacy and sensuality. It awakens your imagination, and sharpens and clarifies your objectives in life.

IT ADDRESSES: Slackened skin, diarrhea, cellulite, water retention, a low libido, scar tissue, eczema, acne, fungal infections, herpes, varicose veins, aggression, mood swings, a temperamental nature, anxiety, tension.

IT HELPS PROMOTE: Groundedness, arousal, certainty, assurance, restoration, persistence, deep relaxation and peace, toned skin, a healthy immune system, weight reduction, cell regeneration, healing.

SAFETY INFORMATION: Nontoxic; not irritating or sensitizing.

PEPPERMINT (mentha piperita)

Peppermint, with its strong and piercing aroma, is one of the most widely and commonly used of all the essential oils, and is native to Europe. It is now also cultivated in Japan and the USA. It grows profusely, with hairy serrated leaves and purple spiked flowers. Its menthol content is used in many medicinal and culinary applications.

The ancient Romans would crown themselves with Peppermint at feasts to take advantage of its detoxifying effects and digestive qualities. The Hebrews said that Peppermint contained aphrodisiac properties; whereas in ancient Greece and Rome, it was considered an everyday part of life—used to scent bath waters, powders, cosmetics, and bed linens.

Medicinally, it is an effective oil, as it expels built-up gas from the digestive tract and is an excellent tonic for the nerves. It is a recovery oil—refreshing the spirit with its potent and sharp effect on the senses, raising attentiveness and awareness, and permeating any environment with its freshness.

As a stimulating oil, first it has a warming effect on the body, and then it cools and refreshes. It energizes, promotes circulation, stimulates the nervous system

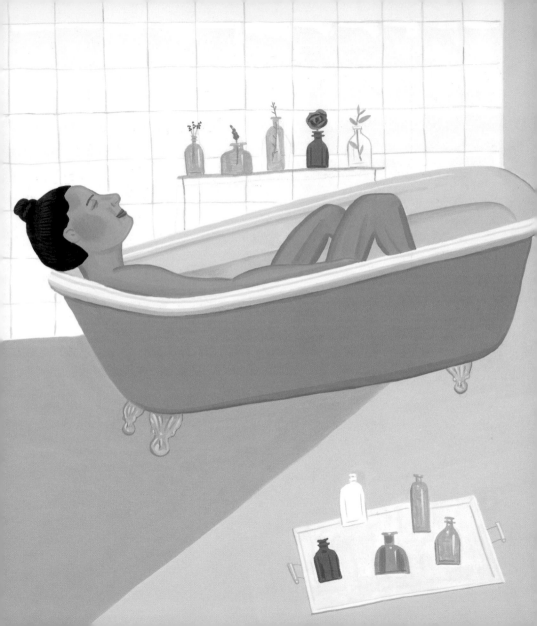

and the brain, and has a potent anti-infectious quality when applied to the body—helping to combat coughs, colds, flus, sore throats, and headaches. With its purifying and decongestant action, it increases the body's capacity to take in oxygen and simultaneously purify the blood.

Peppermint blends well with Eucalyptus and Lemongrass to release muscular aches and pains in the neck and shoulder area, specifically when this pain is associated with stress and nervous conditions. It detoxifies connective tissue, and is therefore of great benefit in sciatica and neuralgia. Due to its numbing effect, it addresses nerve pain and is also beneficial for faintness, giddiness, or lightheadedness.

For areas of the body that have experienced paralysis or numbness, Peppermint acts as a tonic to energize and awaken the nervous system and the senses.

In conjunction with Clary Sage and Basil, it can be used for irregular menstruation and painful periods.

Where any system in the body is weak, use Peppermint to refresh, tone, and bring back vitality—specifically in the intestinal and respiratory systems. Peppermint is by far the most effective of all the essential oils for the digestive system, as it increases its activity and capacity.

It is an excellent oil to use for concentration and for study application, as it prevents nervous exhaustion and overload. Peppermint sharpens the senses, focuses the mind, and can help you absorb new information, allowing you to process effectively while learning.

Peppermint is the oil to use to encourage the digestion of new experiences, while gaining insight and vision into your potential for the future. It engages your attention and purifies thought.

IT ADDRESSES: Asthma, bronchitis, chest infections, sciatica, neuralgia, arthritis, muscular aches and pains, body congestion, flatulence, vomiting, indigestion, colic, diarrhea, liver fatigue, painful menstruation, toothaches, congested skin, mental fatigue, apathy, low vitality, physical exhaustion.

IT HELPS PROMOTE: Regeneration, refreshment, concentration, vitality, energy, enthusiasm, vibrancy, stimulation, clarity, alertness, pain relief, a clear mind and body, good digestion.

SAFETY INFORMATION: Nontoxic, nonirritating. Possible allergic reactions on highly sensitive skin—use in moderation.

Dill +

PETITGRAIN (Citrus aurantium)

Petitgrain oil is produced from the same tree as both Neroli and Orange oil. This specific oil is processed from the leaves and twigs of the bitter orange tree, which is found mainly in the Mediterranean area and primarily grown in France, Italy, North Africa, and Tunisia. Petitgrain, due to its unusual woody and floral bouquet, is used widely throughout the perfume industry as a classic ingredient in eau de colognes. It is pale yellow in color, and has an uplifting quality when used in body-rub blends.

For excessive perspiration, combine it with Cypress oil for an excellent antiperspirant. It is a skin tonic and helps clear up skin blemishes or pimples. Due to its soft bouquet and its anti-infectious properties, it is beneficial when blended with Tea Tree and Lavender for treating acne conditions, boils, and dry skin.

Petitgrain is primarily used as a sedating and calming oil for the nervous system, and its relaxing properties help those suffering from chronic anxiety and insomnia. It assists in breathing and opens the chest to oxygenate the body. When used with Eucalyptus and Cedarwood, it is great for the respiratory system. It is also a digestive stimulant, especially where the nervous system is impeding the digestive processes.

When overcome with anger or feeling emotionally out of control,

Petitgrain restores and brings about renewed insight into prevailing conditions. It stimulates inner vision, strength, and an ability to stabilize; therefore, it encourages open expression. This is an oil to use to dissipate disappointment, release anger, and bring optimism back into your life. Old barriers can melt away, and creativity and communication is allowed to flow. Also, defenses are dropped, and you are left with feelings of joy.

IT ADDRESSES: Acne, boils, dry skin, excessive perspiration, respiratory infections, nervous asthma, muscle spasms, inflammation, arthritis, palpitations, painful digestion, slackened muscles, insomnia, nervous exhaustion, fatigue, anger, frustration.

IT HELPS PROMOTE: Harmony, revival of mind and body, relaxation, sound sleep, insight, stability, good digestion, cardiovascular system, cell regeneration, balance in the nervous system.

SAFETY INFORMATION: Nontoxic; not irritating or sensitizing. It is not phototoxic—even though it is expressed from a citrus tree, it is not from the peel of the fruit.

PINE (Pinus sylvestris)

This tall, inspiring evergreen is found mainly in Northern Europe and can grow to a height of up to 130 feet. The essential oil is taken from the pine's needlelike, gray-green leaves. There are more than 100 species of conifers, and of these, Scotch pine is known for its fresh forest fragrance. It is native to Northern Europe and Russia and grows profusely in North America. This Pine is inspiring and invigorating, reaching lofty heights and exuding a potent aroma that clears the lungs and oxygenates the body.

In ancient times, Pine was used by the Egyptians, the Greeks, and the Arabians, who acknowledged its medicinal properties and used it for pulmonary and chest infections. It has also been associated with religious and spiritual ceremonies, where people bathed in it to purge their bodies.

Pine oil has a potent anti-infectious and anti-microbial effect on the body, helping to create ease of breath for asthmatic, bronchial, and flu-like conditions. In conjunction with

Eucalyptus and Tea Tree, it is an excellent inhalant for sinusitis, sore throats, and laryngitis, as it purifies the sinus passages and the entire respiratory tract. It stimulates circulation and helps excrete debris from the lungs following coughs, colds, and chest complaints.

Pine is an excellent remedy for rheumatoid arthritis, as it eases rheumatic and arthritic pain, gout, and symptoms of sciatica. When blended with Juniper and Cypress, it can be used to relieve water retention and joint stiffness in the body.

Because it energizes and activates, Pine helps increase the metabolic processes of the body and acts as a powerful immune system stimulant. It alleviates the symptoms of colds and flus as it works to address inflammation in the body.

As an antiviral oil, it is excellent when used in conjunction with Niaouli and Myrrh as a topical application. You can use it as a preventive measure during the colder months to keep viruses at bay, and if congestion already exists in the body, it acts as a potent expectorant, cleansing infection and clearing the pathway for oxygen uptake.

When feeling fatigued and lethargic, Pine serves to bring a new sense of vibrancy and vitality to the body. It's fortifying, and it can have a pronounced effect on your vital energy. As it helps to expand the lungs, it opens the chest, which symbolizes opening up your life. It awakens your instinctive nature.

Pine is an oil for protection, and because it inspires and revitalizes you, it is beneficial when feeling weak or suffering from lack of confidence and self-esteem. Pine reminds you that your spirit is the source of inspiration and that it is totally unlimited. It encourages you to trust in yourself and to not be misled or troubled by those around you.

IT ADDRESSES: Infections, congested skin, restricted breathing, asthma, bronchitis, sinusitis, whooping cough, laryngitis, lack of circulation, muscular aches and pains, arthritis, rheumatism, water retention, stiffness, low immunity, coughs, colds, fever, urinary tract infections, debilitation, physical exhaustion, low self-esteem, low energy, nervous exhaustion, fatigue.

IT HELPS PROMOTE: Energy, vitality, vibrancy, mindfulness, certainty, inspiration, direction, a rosy complexion, oxygen uptake, mobility, circulation, a healthy immune system.

SAFETY INFORMATION: Nontoxic, nonirritating. Possible sensitization. Do not use on allergic skin conditions. Do not use during pregnancy.

ROSE (Rosa damascena)

This small shrub is hardy, deciduous, and bushy. It grows to a height of approximately six feet. Rose is a most popular essential oil and has been used for centuries for its sensual aroma and healing qualities. Rosa damascena is cultivated in the Balkan Mountains in Southern Bulgaria, an area known as the "Valley of the Roses." It is also grown in Turkey and France, with similar types being cultivated in China, India, and Russia. This plant is picked right at sunrise to maximize its oil yield, and it takes approximately 20,000 pounds of rose petals to produce one pound of rose oil.

Rose has long been a symbol of love, purity, and trust; it has always been used to heal the heart. In ancient times, the petals were collected for weddings to ensure a prosperous marriage. Rudolf Steiner spoke of the rose's flower, leaf, and root structure being in perfect balance.

Rose is primarily used for the cardiovascular and nervous system. Symbolically, Rose is reputed to reinforce a sense of confidence, self-acceptance, and willpower. It has a tonic effect on the heart, and activates a sluggish metabolism and poor circulation, addressing any cardiac symptoms.

It is generally for people whose immune system is low and where infection is heightened due to long-term anxiety and depression. When the body is stagnant and cold, Rose improves and mobilizes its energy flow. It has an antispasmodic effect on sprains, strains, and chest conditions associated with spasmodic coughing such as bronchitis, coughs, and colds. With its antiviral properties, it protects and strengthens the immune system. It also works to lower high blood pressure, and promotes circulation during recovery from illness. In conjunction with Neroli oil, it can also be used to calm heart palpitations.

Due to its mobilizing qualities, especially in the uterine and reproductive areas of the body, Rose mobilizes stagnant energy that has contributed to irregular or painful menstruation. Therefore, it acts as an excellent tonic for the womb, simultaneously having a calming effect on premenstrual tension. It is good for fertility, increasing self-esteem, and helping with sexual difficulties, specifically in conjunction with frigidity and impotency.

It is particularly beneficial for healing a toxic liver.

Rose oil is the healer of the heart. Where there are old wounds, or feelings of rejection and loss, it restores a sense of comfort and self-worth, and reestablishes your connection to loved ones.

love, gro
calm, inne

It addresses: Urinary infections, cystitis, irregular or painful menstruation, impotency, frigidity, sterility, an inflamed bladder, liver congestion, diarrhea, bronchial disorders, coughs, colds, sprains, strains, palpitations, high blood pressure, broken capillaries, dry and sensitive skin, bitterness, anger, resentment, fear of intimacy, lack of will.

It helps promote: Deep relaxation, love, growth, trust, self-acceptance, nurturing, forgiveness, inner peace, soft and silky skin, a refined and rosy complexion, a balanced menstrual cycle, healthy female reproductive organs, strength of the heart.

Safety information: Nontoxic, nonirritating. Do not use on highly sensitive skin.

ROSEMARY (Rosmarinus officinalis)

This traditional herb, commonly used for medicinal and culinary purposes, is one of the oldest documented herbs, and is distilled from the flowering tops of the plant. Its woody stems can grow up to three feet tall and exhibit a blue-lilac flower. It is native to Asian countries, and is also found widely throughout the Mediterranean region. The essential oil is produced in France, Tunisia, and Yugoslavia.

When Egyptian tombs were opened, Rosemary was found in them, and it was said to have been buried as a symbol of regeneration. In ancient times, gods were adorned with sprigs of Rosemary, and it was used in ceremonial procedures to banish evil spirits. Rosemary was widely used during plagues due to its reputation for guarding against negative energy, and also for its medicinal value, as it protects the body from infection.

Rosemary's stimulating and activating properties were revered in skin care; it was said to restore vitality and youth. These ancient uses of the herb probably contributed to Rosemary being considered one of the most versatile oils for stimulating and invigorating the body and mind.

Rosemary is said to revive the memory and help with recall. It is an excellent revitalizing tonic, as it stimulates circulation, activates metabolism, and provides the body with energy and vitality.

Rosemary combats physical and mental lethargy, and strengthens arterial blood flow. It elevates low blood pressure and promotes circulation to the extremities of the body. It is especially useful during the colder months when nervous debility is experienced due to poor circulation and concentration.

In combination with Eucalyptus and Juniper, it makes an excellent sports rub. During exercise, it assists blood flow, therefore acting against the buildup of lactic acid after training. It is an antirheumatic oil, and in conditions of cold or cramping, it alleviates muscular stiffness, sprains, and strains.

Rosemary is a decongestant, expectorant, restorative, stimulant, and general body tonic, especially useful when the body is feeling debilitated. Rosemary is also a liver decongestant; and is beneficial for conditions such as cirrhosis of the liver, gallstones, bile duct blockage, and hepatitis.

Rosemary also has a mild diuretic property, which helps with water retention, especially during menstruation and menopause. It assists with weight loss, as it promotes a balanced metabolism and helps the body break down fats. It revives the senses and plays an active role in restoring balance to the central nervous system.

It is excellent to use following paralysis; or where cramps, strains, sprains, or degeneration of muscular tissue has occurred in the body.

Rosemary is a tonic for the skin, easing congestion and reducing puffiness and swelling. It can be used as a hair stimulant; and in conjunction with Tea Tree and Cedarwood, it helps control dandruff.

Rosemary helps you build confidence and morale. It establishes greater awareness of your own potential and reminds you of your inner self. It reconnects you to your purpose and stimulates clarity and intention, thereby helping you move forward.

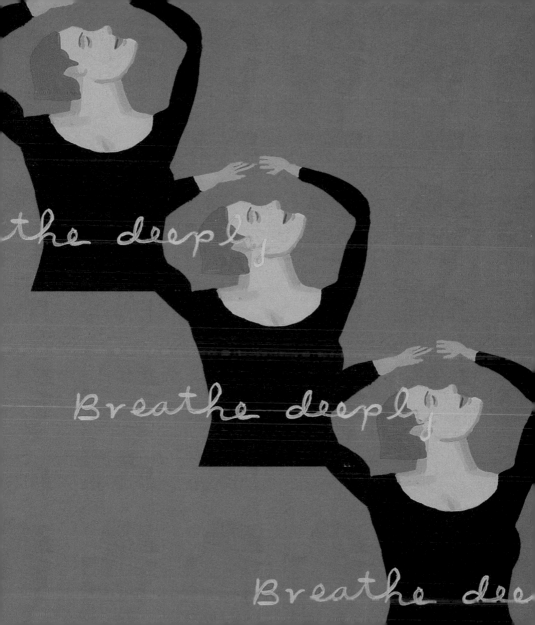

IT ADDRESSES: Respiratory infections, congestion, bronchitis, sinusitis, rheumatism, muscular aches and pains, paralysis, sprains, poor circulation, low blood pressure, headaches, flatulence, constipation, slow metabolism, a sluggish liver, edema, obesity, cellulite, nervous exhaustion, migraines, poor memory, lethargy, impediments to the senses, feeling overwhelmed or overtired, poor memory, lack of focus.

IT HELPS PROMOTE: Energy, vitality, sharpening of the senses, promotion of a healthy ego, concentration, memory, hair growth, venous flow, circulation, strength to the chest, muscle tone, elimination of toxins, a healthy cardiovascular system, regeneration, toned skin, weight loss.

SAFETY INFORMATION: Nontoxic; not irritating or sensitizing. Do not use on traumatized or damaged skin. Do not use if there's high blood pressure. Do not use during pregnancy. Do not use with epileptics.

ROSEWOOD (Aniba roseaodora)

This evergreen tree, which grows to almost 130 feet tall, is found in the tropical rain forest of South America. The distillation of this woody and floral oil is largely obtained from the wood chips of the tree's heartwood.

Rosewood's medicinal properties are said to influence on more of a psychological level than on a physical level. It is a remedy for the immune system, said to boost and refresh a capacity to fight viruses and bacteria. On an emotional level, it brings stability to the central nervous system; therefore, it has a balancing effect on nervous conditions for those who feel overworked.

Rosewood helps calm the mind during meditation and is excellent to use during travel, as it assists in restabilizing the body, acting as a preventive measure against jet lag.

It is an aphrodisiac; and also brings a sense of warmth, peace, and security to those who have suffered from sexual abuse.

On the skin, Rosewood is excellent for inflammations and allergies. It also helps combat wrinkles and premature aging, due to its ability to stimulate cell regeneration in the tissue.

Rosewood has anti-infectious and anti-viral attributes, addressing bronchial and pulmonary infections, especially in young children and babies. It is a muscle tonic, and can therefore be used after exercise and during weight-loss programs.

Rosewood has a gentle and calming influence on the body, and is particularly beneficial in a warm bath at the end of the day. It allows you to be mindful of future possibilities and lulls you into a gentle slumber.

It addresses: Dry, sensitive, inflamed skin; dermatitis scars; premature aging; wrinkles; bronchial infections; headaches; nausea (particularly during travel); inflammations; depression; insecurity; uncertainty; nervous tension.

It helps promote: Regeneration to the skin and nervous system, warmth and balance, energy, peace, relaxation, muscle tone, stability, balance to the central nervous system.

Safety information: Nontoxic; not irritating or sensitizing. Use with caution on allergic-prone skin.

SAGE (Salvia officinalis)

This hardy evergreen shrub, a native of Southern Europe, has a clear, sharp aroma. Sage has gray-green leaves and tubular blue flowers. It tends to grow almost two feet high, and grows wild in Yugoslavia and Dalmatia. Ideally, though, Sage oil is extracted from plants grown in the Mediterranean region.

The ancient Chinese believed that Sage was a cure for sterility. The Greeks used it in herbal remedies to combat liver disease.

Sage is praised today for its capacity to deal with women's

physical disorders; it acts as a tonic, stimulating the reproductive organs. It is beneficial as a blood purifier and cleanser, and is excellent to use when fatigue overrides the body and weakness and debility are apparent. For those who are running hard in life's marathon, trying to keep all the balls juggling, Sage helps maintain momentum. It increases energy, is an emotional purifier, and clears the way for the expression of wisdom.

Sage has a cleansing effect on the lymphatic system and liver, and also aids the digestive system. Those suffering from loss of appetite or constipation often find it beneficial; it is particularly useful after the consumption of a heavy meal, as it cleanses and stimulates the digestive tract. It has the ability to regulate fluids in the body and works to combat water retention and edema.

Sage clears congestion in the body and is excellent for heavy sweating during menstruation and menopause.

Acting as an astringent, Sage tightens and tones the skin, decongesting and cleansing dirty and clogged pores. This is the oil to use to accelerate skin metabolism and give a soft, feminine glow to your complexion.

Sage helps create mobility in the body. When heading to the gym, make sure Sage is packed for an after-sport body

GERAnium for harmony, balance, security, comfort, regularity in menstrual cycle.

rub, since it increases the delivery of energy to the body's cells, as well as functioning as an antiperspirant.

Sage acts as a rescue oil when you're feeling emotionally overwhelmed and fragile; it reassures you, and assists in redirecting vital energies throughout the body, taking the focus away from that out-of-control feeling. Overall, it allows for inner growth and strength.

It addresses:

Congestion due to colds, bronchitis, respiratory disorders (especially with excess fluid), cold sores, ulcers, dermatitis, oily or sweaty skin, hair loss, rheumatoid arthritis, muscle aches and pains, low blood pressure, excess bleeding, a sluggish immune system, viral infections, liver disorders, menstrual irregularities, menopausal sweating, migraines, depression, mental strain, physical exhaustion, grief, weepy emotional states, helplessness.

IT HELPS PROMOTE: Sensory acuity, improved memory, a purified mind, expanded wisdom, regeneration, a balanced cycle, an energized digestive system, a cleansed liver, a healthy immune system, regulated fluids in the body.

SAFETY INFORMATION: Not irritating or sensitizing. In excess, it may overwhelm the nervous system. Do not use if you're epileptic. Do not use during pregnancy. Avoid use with babies and young children. Should be avoided by nursing mothers.

SANDALWOOD (Santalum album)

Sandalwood is a small evergreen parasitic tree that grows to a height of 30 feet. The essential oil is extracted from the heartwood of the tree, which is chopped and chipped for distillation. The tree has leathery leaves and slender branches and is usually more than 30

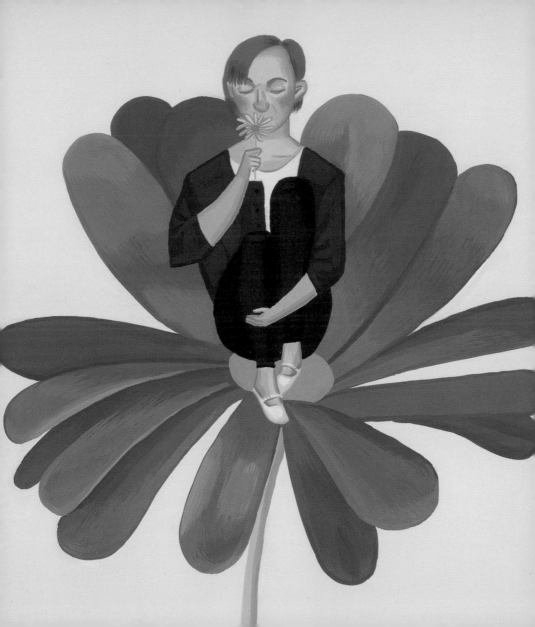

years old before it is harvested for extraction. It is native to Southern Asia, and most of the world's Sandalwood oil is grown and extracted in the Mysore region of India. Sandalwood is also grown in Australia, but it is not known to have any medicinal or therapeutic value.

For hundreds of years, Sandalwood has been used for sacred, medicinal, and religious purposes. The ancient Egyptians used Sandalwood to embalm, and in ritual and religious ceremonies, to venerate the gods. In Ayurvedic (Indian) medicine, dating back hundreds of years, Sandalwood was used for its potent anti-infectious qualities and renowned for its ability to treat mind and body simultaneously.

On the body, Sandalwood acts as an astringent to heal skin inflammation; and it has a potent ability to clear intestinal, genital, and urinary disorders. In conjunction with Lavender and Tea Tree, its cooling effect makes it an excellent oil to use to treat cystitis or inflammation of the kidney area.

Sandalwood also has the capacity to soothe and strengthen the chest area, and is recommended for respiratory infections such as bronchitis. Combined with an oxygenating oil such as Eucalyptus, it can be used to soothe irritation and inflammation, and open the respiratory pathways. To treat sore throats, use

Sandalwood with Clary Sage.

Sandalwood strengthens the skin's connective tissues, as it increases capillary circulation. Used in a compress with Chamomile, it heals areas that have been traumatized or subjected to severe weather conditions. Sandalwood helps ease skin inflammations; and relieves eczema, dermatitis, abscesses, or cracks and fissures caused by overexposure to harsh environments or nervous conditions.

Sandalwood instills a deep sense of tranquility in people. It is an excellent oil to use during meditation or when you want to create alignment with a loved one, as it dissipates the worry of everyday life and gives you the opportunity to reinvest yourself intimately into the relationship. It is an oil for courage and confidence, bringing about a sense of groundedness in the face of rapid change.

Sandalwood is revered for its capacity to encourage gestation of new ideas and creativity, allowing space for change and growth. It creates a path to peace.

> **IT ADDRESSES:** Infections, acne, oily skin, chafed or weakened skin, congestion, bronchitis, dry coughs, laryngitis, sore throats, muscular spasms, diarrhea, urinary tract infections, kidney inflammations, rigidity, impotency, depression, insomnia, stress, aggression, grief.

IT HELPS PROMOTE: Warmth, courage, serenity, unity, one-ness, sensuality, acceptance, groundedness, security, skin regeneration, good cardiac function, muscle ease, improved kidney function, enhanced hormonal and reproductive functions.

SAFETY INFORMATION: Nontoxic; not irritating or sensitizing.

SPIKENARD (Nardostachys Jatamansi)

Spikenard, native to the mountainous areas of Northern India, China, and Japan, is one of the most ancient of all the aromatic substances. A tender herb with a pungent fragrance, it grows to a height of approximately three feet, exuding small green flowers. The oil itself is extracted from the fragrant root system, which gives Spikenard its inherent quality of stability.

One of its main functions in herbal and folk tradition is as a diuretic. In ancient texts, Spikenard is depicted as an oil for both ritual and medicinal applications. It was pounded into an ointment and used to anoint the feet of Christ, for its intrinsic healing qualities. It is closely associated with the attributes of Frankincense and Myrrh, acknowledged for their associations with the spirit.

Spikenard's use as a perfume was well documented in ancient Greek texts, where it was applied in preparations as a balm for the body and soul. Use this oil to regulate and sustain you.

Spikenard's capacity to stabilize body, mind, and emotions while restoring rhythmic balance is of great benefit when addressing nervous tension, anxiety, and insomnia. It is highly recommended for the venous system and for treating disorders such as hemorrhoids and varicose veins. It enhances blood flow in the genital area, the urinary tract, and the reproductive organs, especially the ovaries. It is also good for anemia.

Of great benefit to the digestive tract, Spikenard oil serves to mobilize and dissipate any constriction that occurs, such as flatulence and constipation. Like all root oils, it has the capacity to dig deep into the subcutaneous tissue and regenerate cells. Spikenard restores your spirit, connecting you to a deep inner peace.

Spikenard embraces the heart, stabilizes the mind, and restores the emotions. It can balance out feelings of urgency, which often take you off your true path. This oil encourages you to be at peace with yourself.

IT ADDRESSES: Allergies, rashes, psoriasis, inflammations, wounds, prematurely aging skin, hair loss, hemorrhoids, varicose veins, thrombosis, an irregular heartbeat, sluggish circulation, constipation, indigestion, physical and emotional exhaustion, insomnia, despondency, struggles, lack of purpose.

IT HELPS PROMOTE: Compassion, wisdom, healing, spiritual certainty, devotion, balance, emotional poise, a spiritual/physical connection, clear skin, strengthened and regenerated tissue, healthy lung function, good circulation.

SAFETY INFORMATION: Nontoxic; not irritating or sensitizing. Do not use during pregnancy, or with babies and young children under age five.

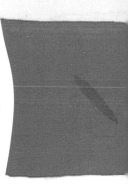

SPEARMINT (mentha spicata)

Spearmint is a hardy perennial herb with flowering tops. It has a bright green leaf with a sweet mint aroma, and sheds pink-lilac flowers. This oil is predominantly produced in the USA, Hungary, Spain, Yugoslavia, Russia, and China. It is also grown throughout Northern Africa, and grows wild in Morocco. It is native to the Mediterranean region and grows throughout the Middle East. There are many different types of mint, and it is widely utilized medicinally, cosmetically, and for culinary purposes.

181

The ancient Greeks used Spearmint as a restorative agent for the body. It was used aromatically in the bathwater prior to sleep, as a digestive aid. Applied to the forehead and temple, Spearmint is said to alleviate an overworked and overburdened mind.

Spearmint is an excellent oil to use with young children for its sweet smell, and healing and restorative qualities. Being much milder than its relative, Peppermint, it is great for children's disorders, as it is less potent, yet equally effective.

Spearmint has an antispasmodic effect on muscles and the chest, as it opens and refreshes the respiratory pathway. In a bath, the aromatic waters invigorate the senses and soothe the muscles. It is excellent when massaged onto the abdominal area to treat flatulence and disorders of the digestive tract.

Spearmint provides a refreshing tonic to the skin, since it cleanses the pores and refreshes the complexion. This oil brings any entertainment environment alive; it helps move conversation along and promotes improved food digestion. Refreshing and energizing, it makes a great dinner companion.

With its fresh mint aroma, Spearmint is the oil to use to bring comfort to the mind and ease to the body, particularly when you're busy digesting life. It brings about increased awareness and an almost childlike innocence. It is stimulating and activating, inspiring clarity and lightness during times of mental exhaustion.

IT ADDRESSES: Congestion due to colds, colic, dyspepsia, flatulence, nausea, vomiting (especially in children), dermatitis conditions, processing problems, loss of clarity and insight, lethargy.

IT HELPS PROMOTE: Lightheartedness, awareness, innocence, clarity, energy cleansing, ease of menstruation, a healthy appetite, good digestion, strength of the chest, clean skin.

SAFETY INFORMATION: Nontoxic; not irritating or sensitizing.

TEA TREE (melaleuca alternifolia)

This small tree with narrow leaves grows to a height of approximately 20 feet and flourishes in its native home of Australia. Its flowers are yellow and shaped like bottle brushes, and the essential oil is extracted from its needle-like leaves. Due to its anti-infectious qualities, Tea Tree has been used as an herbal tea to prevent disease and various disorders. It is one of the most potent oils for treating bacteria, viruses, and fungal infections.

Whenever the body is threatened by bacteria, use Tea Tree as a preventive measure to strengthen and protect. While Tea Tree has been used for its pungent aroma and as a remedy for colds, coughs, flus, and

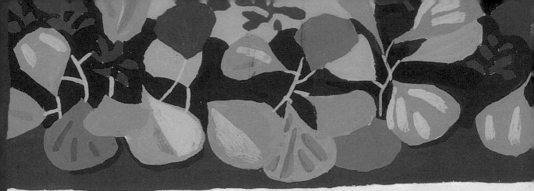

headaches, it was not until after World War I that the plant's specific medical applications were identified. Tea Tree was found to be 12 times stronger than the medications being administered at the time.

Tea Tree's antiseptic capacity in the treatment of bacterial infections is remarkable. As a result, it is one of the most powerful disinfectants, and being one of the most non-irritating of all the essential oils, it is highly valued as a natural antibiotic.

Tea Tree permeates and kills invading organisms in the body as it stimulates your system. It has a wide application in the treatment of viral and fungal infections, and strengthens the body's resistance, thereby preventing the recurrence of the infection.

Tea Tree can be used to address a wide range of respiratory ailments, and works with most other oils to effectively cleanse the body and strengthen the lungs. It is a powerful tonic when applied topically to the body in a massage blend to detoxify and energize.

It stimulates circulation, and in cases of emergency can be used to disinfect and cleanse wounds, burns, and bites. It also treats fungal infections such as athlete's foot, thrush, mouth ulcers, any mucous membrane condition, and other body infections. It is an excellent first-aid oil.

Tea Tree can also be used to treat disorders where discharge is apparent, such as dandruff, vaginitis, and weeping sores.

For those with a delicate physical disposition, Tea Tree fortifies and protects. On an emotional level, this oil cleanses toxic emotions that can eventually undermine the health and well-being of the body.

IT ADDRESSES: Abscesses, acne, athlete's foot, cold sores, insect bites, wounds, infections, dermatitis, asthma, bronchitis, congestion, colds, coughs, fevers, flus, sinusitis, whooping cough, thrush, vaginitis, cystitis, lethargy, debility, vulnerability, shallow breathing.

IT HELPS PROMOTE: Stability; energy and vitality; strength; good circulation; blood flow to the brain; protection against infections; anti-bacterial, anti-inflammatory, and anti-fungal actions.

SAFETY INFORMATION: Nontoxic, nonsensitizing. Possible skin irritant in high doses.

THYME
(Thymus vulgaris)

Thyme is a strong perennial shrub, growing to a height of approximately 1 ½ feet. With its gray-green leaf and small white-to-lilac flowers, it is most commonly found in Mediterranean regions. It is produced in Spain, France, Greece, and Morocco. In more recent times, it has also been produced in Asia, Algeria, Turkey, Tunisia, Israel, the USA, Russia, and China.

Traditionally, Thyme was used by the ancient Greeks to fumigate environments against infections and the onslaught of disease. The ancient Roman soldiers would bathe in Thyme before entering battle to raise morale and bring about enhanced focus and energy. It is well known for its culinary applications, specifically its use in preserving meats. The Egyptians knew about this preserving quality, so they would use Thyme in the embalming process. Today it still has a wide range of uses in herbal medicine, mostly used for respiratory disorders, digestive complaints, and the prevention of disease.

Thyme is one of the most potent antimicrobial oils and is an excellent antioxidant; therefore, it can be used to promote longevity. Its strong herbaceous aroma indicates that it has qualities to drive, energize, and encourage you.

This powerful tonic for the body reinforces the functions of the lungs, heart, kidneys, and nervous system. Where any condition of weakness arises in the body due to infection, congestion, or debilitation, Thyme stimulates the body into action. It is also used to promote regeneration in sleep and to revive and strengthen the body and mind.

Thyme can clear the lungs of congestion and inflammation, and helps relieve bronchial conditions.

In conjunction with the toning action of Rosemary, Thyme strengthens the circulatory system. It can also be used as a potent digestive aid, to revive low spirits, and to overcome feelings of exhaustion. It raises low blood pressure and is excellent for arthritis, rheumatism, and sciatica. Its stimulating effect and diuretic action assist in the removal of uric acid from the body when applied topically in a body-rub blend.

Thyme is an excellent tonic for sluggish systems, as it fortifies and uplifts body and mind. This oil can help you harness your energy and give you the strength to forge ahead in life. It takes courage and drive to fulfill your passions—Thyme encourages natural enthusiasm and dynamism to help you get back into the swing of things.

IT ADDRESSES: Acne, oily skin, scalp disorders, sinusitis, pharyngitis, bronchitis, pneumonia, arthritis, neuromuscular disorders, poor circulation, infections, indigestion, tonsillitis, endometriosis, nervous exhaustion, stress, mental fatigue, debilitation, withdrawal, despondency and low morale, apprehension.

IT HELPS PROMOTE: Revival, courage, forging forward, physical and emotional strength, fortitude, vigor, improved digestion, a healthy immune system, warmth, balance to the reproductive system, stimulated hormones, good circulation.

SAFETY INFORMATION: Do not use during pregnancy. Do not use with babies or young children under age five. Low irritant, low toxicity. Use in moderation due to its potency. Do not use on mucous membranes.

VETIVER (vetiveria zizanoides)

This tall perennial scented grass grows with a straight stem and narrow leaves. Its abundant root system is pungently fragrant and used for essential oil extraction. In its wild state, Vetiver grows native in Southern India, Indonesia, and Sri Lanka; it is now also cultivated in the Philippines, the

Comoro Islands, West Africa, and South America. It is produced in Java, Haiti, and a small island near Madagascar called Reunion.

The exotic, earthy fragrance of Vetiver has been used for centuries during India's hot summers, as it helps to hydrate the environment. For this reason, it is also used as an insect repellent. In both India and Java, Vetiver is known as the oil of tranquility.

While Vetiver is botanically related to Lemongrass, Citronella, and Palmarosa, it is more often used for inflammatory disorders of the joints, rheumatoid arthritis, and skin conditions such as eczema. Its cool and potent energy qualifies it as an antiseptic and antispasmodic oil. It purges the body and is used as a preventive measure for fevers. It is a sedative to the nervous system, while being a stimulant to the circulatory system.

As with all root oils, Vetiver reflects the deep richness of the earth; therefore, it helps support, restore, absorb, and process.

Vetiver is well known for its capacity to reactivate a poor appetite, disperse nutrients, and assist in weight loss. As it renews the body's strength, it also strengthens and restores the connective tissue, and is excellent for weakness in the joints and undernourished skin.

This hormone tonic is especially beneficial for premenstrual tension and menopausal problems. It is an excellent oil to use in postoperative care. After childbirth, it can help a new mother feel more uplifted.

Vetiver relieves muscular aches and pains, especially those associ-

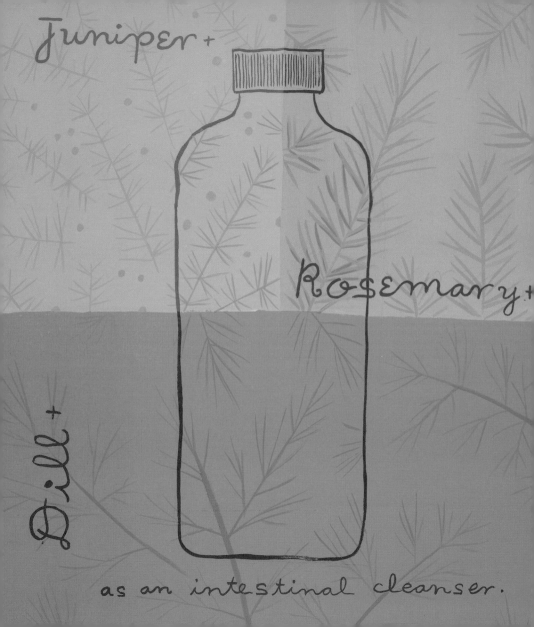

Juniper +

Rosemary +

Dill +

as an intestinal cleanser.

ated with rheumatism and arthritis, bringing about a warm and energetic flow to the body. It is a tonic for the reproductive system and works specifically to reduce tension associated with sexual/sensual expression. When the body is overworked, or when extreme physical, mental, and emotional discipline has been inflicted on the body, Vetiver oil replenishes.

Vetiver restores, revitalizes, and renews, as it reconnects you to a sense of belonging and connection with the earth. It nourishes your soul and replenishes your spirit by allowing you to gently process and digest life's experiences. It is the oil of abundance and has the capacity to reconnect you with universal energy.

IT ADDRESSES: Inflammatory disorders of the joints, rheumatoid arthritis, skin conditions, eczema, fevers, the nervous system and circulatory systems, poor appetite, the connective tissues, pre-menstrual tension, postoperative and postnatal care, disconnection, depression, flagging spirits, lethargy.

IT HELPS PROMOTE: Restoration, revitalization, renewal, connection, balance, comfort, abundance, hydration, cooling, moisture, antiseptic and antispasmodic actions, sedation of the nervous system, stimulation of the circulatory system, cell renewal, tranquility, grounding.

SAFETY INFORMATION: Nontoxic; not irritating or sensitizing.

YLANG YLANG
(Cananga odorata)

This exotic and tropical evergreen can grow up to 65 feet tall, producing shiny oval-shaped leaves and pale green flowers that often turn deep yellow as they mature. The oil is extracted from the Ylang Ylang flower within 24 hours of picking. Similar to the delicate flower of Jasmine, it arouses and has a provocative effect on the senses. Ylang Ylang is native to tropical Asia and is used by the Islanders; it is immersed in coconut oil to produce a pomade that is rubbed over the body to prevent fevers and guard against infection. It is also applied to the hair to nourish and protect.

In Indonesia, the Ylang Ylang flowers were traditionally spread over the beds of newlyweds on their wedding night to arouse them and bring peace to the relationship. Ylang Ylang is a potent aphrodisiac, with the ability to work effectively on impotency and frigidity, while at the same time relaxing the central nervous system and allowing for more confident sexual expression during intimate moments.

It dissipates anger, and as an anti-inflammatory oil, it works effectively on physical and emotional levels. Ylang Ylang balances the reproductive hormones, stimulating and regulating the natural functions of the genito-urinary and reproductive systems.

Oriental medicine, being one of the oldest forms of herbal medicine, attributes to Ylang Ylang a calming and supportive action on the heart and cardiac system.

Ylang Ylang helps calm nervous tension, regulate heartbeat, and dissipate hypertension. It settles restlessness and frustration and encourages sound sleep.

At the U.K.'s Birmingham University, Dr. Tim Betts of the neuropsychiatric clinic reports that Ylang Ylang can influence the onset of an epileptic seizure. In testing the oil, he found that the majority of patients with epilepsy would choose Ylang Ylang almost every time when given a selection of four or five essential oils.

When combined with Clary Sage and Sandalwood, Ylang Ylang can be a provocative blend for an intimate dinner. When feeling withdrawn sexually and wanting to reconnect and relax in intimate environments, Ylang Ylang is the oil to use to arouse and create a euphoric atmosphere. For those who are anxious, Ylang Ylang promotes flow and balance. Its harmonizing effects can help you reconnect with life.

Ylang Ylang is an oil of joy and pleasure—it opens the heart, replenishes the senses, and encourages ecstasy and passion.

IT ADDRESSES: Oily or irritated skin, palpitations, high blood pressure, fever, malaria, intestinal infections, imbalanced hormones, impotency, frigidity, insomnia, nervous tension, inner coldness, anger, low self-esteem.

IT HELPS PROMOTE: Ecstasy, euphoria, creativity, sensuality, inner peace, a passion for life, deep relaxation, arousal, regulation of the adrenals, pleasure during sex, support to the nervous system, harmony.

SAFETY INFORMATION: Do not use on damaged or sensitized skin. Can cause headaches in large doses.

✼ ✼ ✼

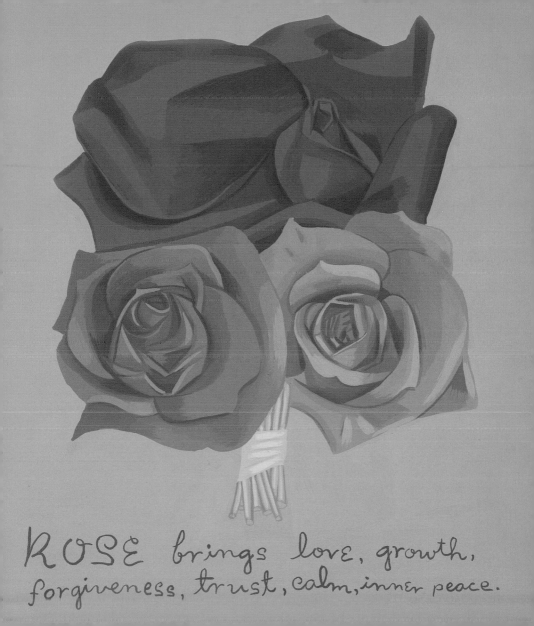

ROSE brings love, growth, forgiveness, trust, calm, inner peace.

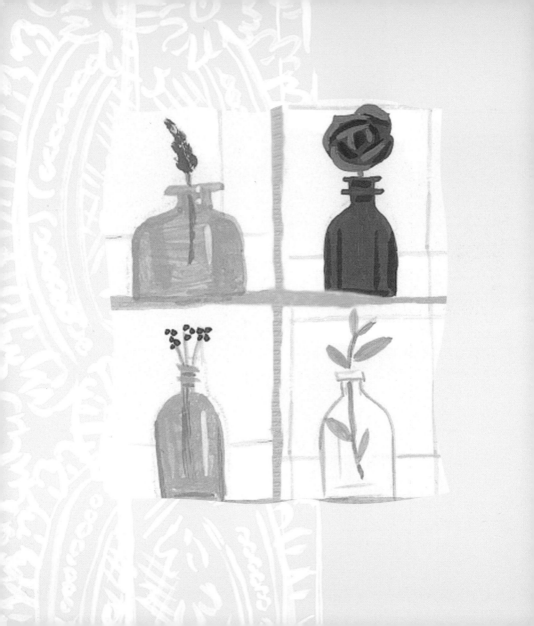

About the Author

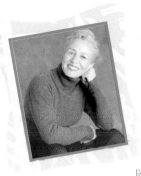

KAREN DOWNES has co-authored five other aromatherapy/lifestyle books, with more than 500,000 copies sold worldwide. She works as an activist with The Hunger Project; and as a consultant travels extensively, conducting lectures and programs that help to empower women to live their lives fully. Karen lives in Melbourne, Australia, with her husband, Jeffrey; and daughter, Rebecca.

Karen can be contacted by e-mail:
downes@netspace.net.au

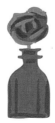

Hay House Lifestyles Titles

Flip Books

101 Ways to Happiness, by Louise L. Hay

101 Ways to Health and Healing, by Louise L. Hay

101 Ways to Romance, by Barbara De Angelis, Ph.D.

101 Ways to Transform Your Life, by Dr. Wayne W. Dyer

Books

A Garden of Thoughts, by Louise L. Hay

Aromatherapy A-Z, by Connie Higley, Alan Higley, and Pat Leatham

Aromatherapy 101, by Karen Downes

Colors & Numbers, by Louise L. Hay

Constant Craving A-Z, by Doreen Virtue, Ph.D.

Dream Journal, by Leon Nacson

Healing with Herbs and Home Remedies A-Z, by Hanna Kroeger

Healing with the Angels Oracle Cards (booklet and card pack), by Doreen Virtue, Ph.D.

Heal Your Body A-Z, by Louise L. Hay

Home Design with Feng Shui A-Z, by Terah Kathryn Collins

Homeopathy A-Z, by Dana Ullman, M.P.H.

Interpreting Dreams A-Z, by Leon Nacson

Natural Gardening A-Z, by Donald W. Trotter, Ph.D.

Natural Healing for Dogs and Cats A-Z, by Cheryl Schwartz, D.V.M.

Natural Pregnancy A-Z, by Carolle Jean-Murat, M.D.

Pleasant Dreams, by Amy E. Dean

Weddings A-Z, by Deborah McCoy

What Color Is Your Personality? by Carol Ritberger, Ph.D.

What Is Spirit?, by Lexie Brockway Potamkin

You Can Heal Your Life, by Louise L. Hay . . . and

Power Thought Cards, by Louise L. Hay (affirmation cards)

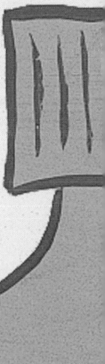

All of the above titles may be ordered by calling Hay House at (760) 431-7695 or (800) 654-5126.

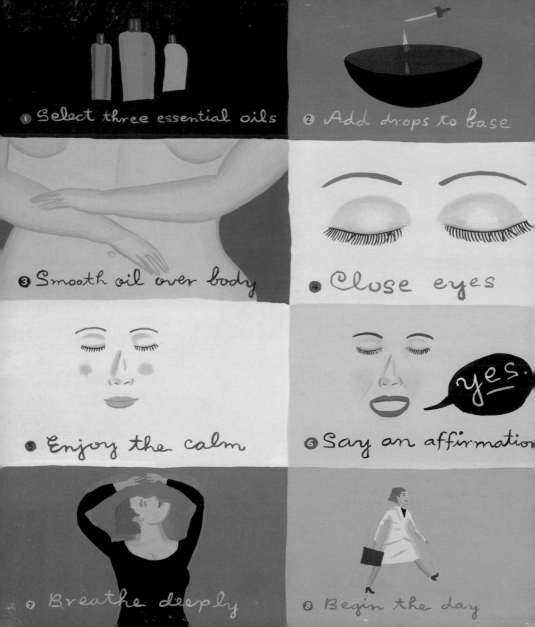

We hope you enjoyed this Hay House Lifestyles book.
If you would like to receive a free catalog featuring additional
Hay House books and products, or if you would like information
about the Hay Foundation, please contact:

Hay House, Inc.
P.O. Box 5100
Carlsbad, CA 92018-5100

(760) 431-7695 or (800) 654-5126
(760) 431-6948 (fax) or (800) 650-5115 (fax)

Please visit the Hay House Website at: www.hayhouse.com

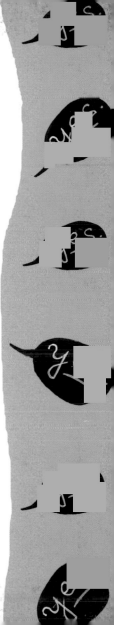

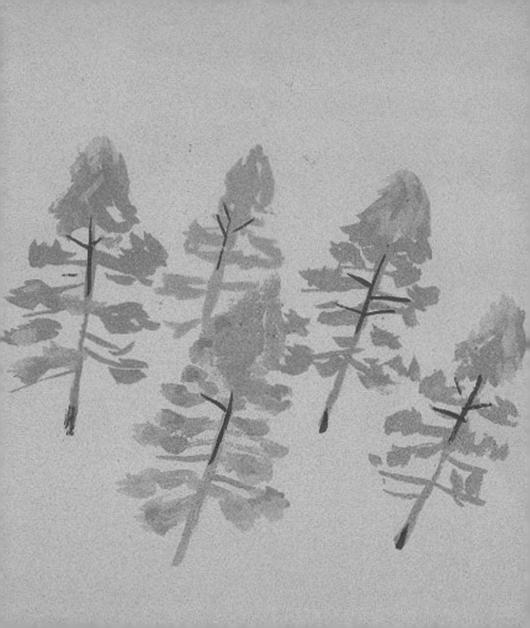

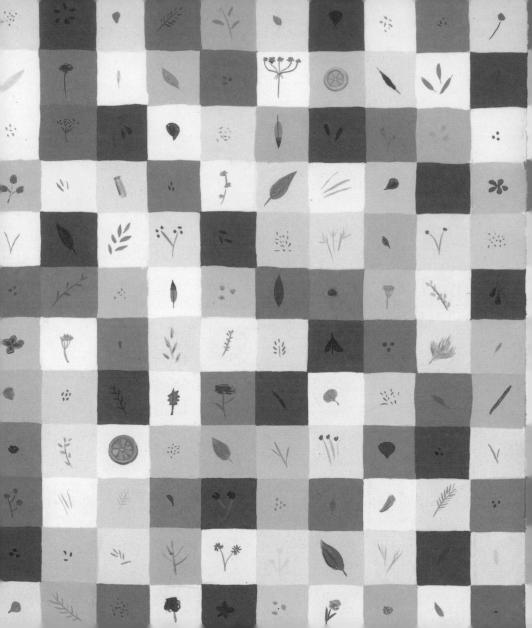